Up and Running

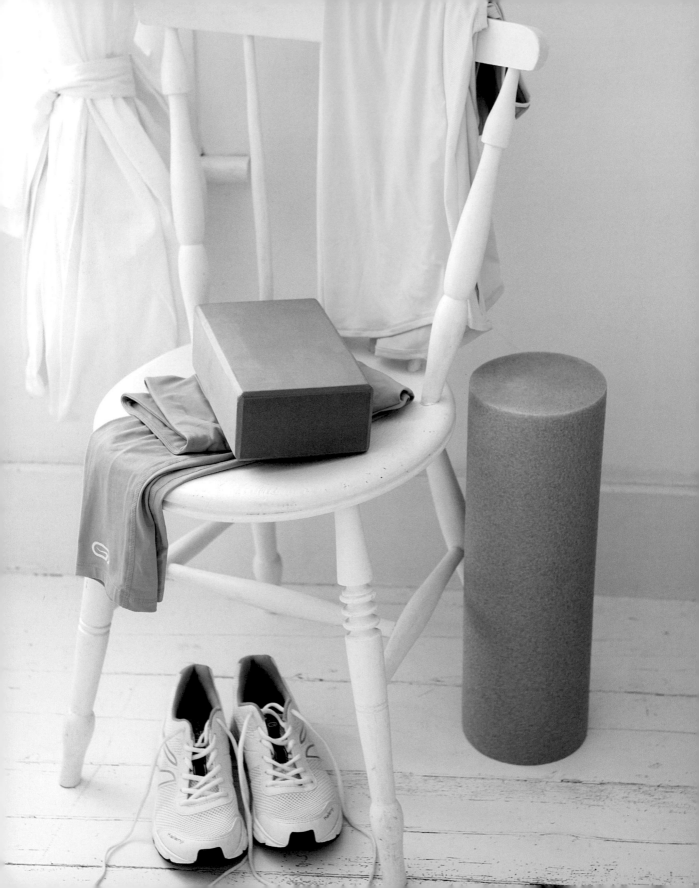

Up and Running

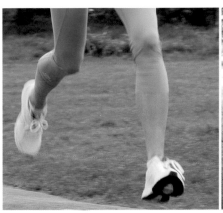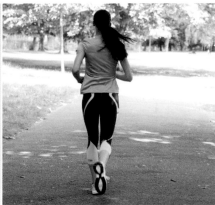

**Your 8-week Plan to go
from 0–5k and beyond and discover the
life-changing power of running!**

Julia Jones and Shauna Reid

Foreword by Bart Yasso

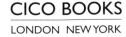

CICO BOOKS
LONDON NEW YORK

To all our Up & Runners around the world.

Published in 2015 by CICO Books
An imprint of Ryland Peters & Small Ltd
20–21 Jockey's Fields, London WC1R 4BW
341 E. 116th Street, New York, NY 10029

www.rylandpeters.com

10 9 8 7 6 5 4 3 2 1

Text © Julia Jones and Shauna Reid 2015
Design and photography © CICO Books 2015

A CIP catalog record for this book is
available from the Library of Congress and
the British Library.

ISBN: 978 1 78249 168 2

Printed in China

Editor: Jennifer Jahn
Designer: Alison Fenton
Photographer: Penny Wincer
Stylist: Isabel de Cordova

Commissioning editor: Lauren Mulholland
In-house designer: Fahema Khanam
Art director: Sally Powell
Production controller: Gordana Simakovic
Publishing manager: Penny Craig
Publisher: Cindy Richards

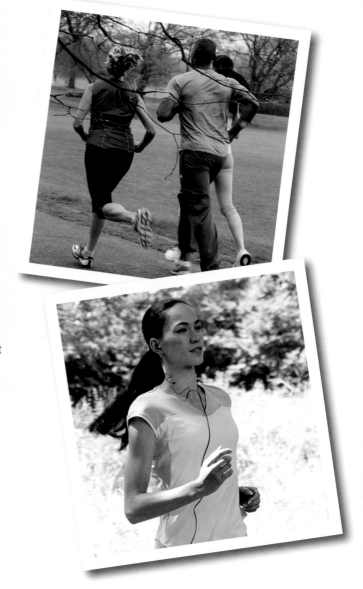

Contents

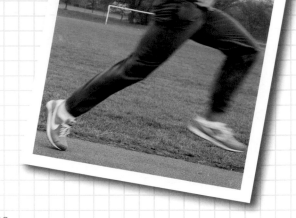

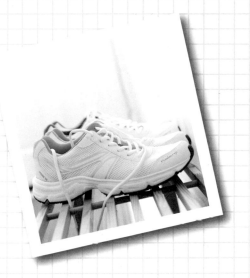

Foreword

My first memories of running are from 1977. I wish I had a picture of me running in my cut-off jeans, cotton t-shirt and crummy sneakers, but back then there were no cellphones to snap a selfie. I was 22 years old and running was booming. Frank Shorter had won the marathon gold medal at the 1972 Olympics and the silver in 1976. Jim Fixx's *The Complete Book of Running* was a smash bestseller. Something sparked my interest and I needed a change because I was not leading a healthy life at that moment. So I just started running, heading out the door with my Collie dog Brandy for a little run…

It was mentally tough at first. I thought, "how can I run if I'm not a runner?" But you've got to start somewhere. Initially I really needed the dog to get me motivated, but once I could cover what felt like a mile, it was time to set out on my own. That's when I knew I was in it for the long haul.

It slowly grew from there. I went to the local track and ran an actual mile, then before I knew it I was doing two or three miles every other day. I gradually built up to comfortably running 30 to 40 miles per week. Then one day, my older brother George challenged me to sign up for a road race. Once I crossed that first finish line, I was hooked.

Running captivates me for many reasons. There's the beauty and the sheer freedom of it. You just go out there and you're in control of everything. Nobody tells you what to feel or what to do. It's a moment with yourself, for yourself. And you can see your progression over time, which is a nice thing.

Racing hooked me too. It's challenging and I like challenges. Most of us aren't out there setting world records or competing for Olympic medals. It's just you against the clock.

The most surprising and powerful reward is being part of the running community. Whether online or offline, it's an accepting and embracing group of people. Once I got into that fold, I flourished. Not only in my running but also in my career and every other facet of my life.

The first thing I say when people ask me how to start running is that everybody is a runner, they just don't know it yet. All you have to do is make that commitment and do it. We always have a perception of what a runner is and worry we don't fit into that mold. But go watch any running race and I promise, you'll see yourself go by. Whether you're 20 or 80, whether you weigh 120 lbs or 300 lbs, you're going to find someone just like you. That's when the lightbulb turns on and you'll think, if they're doing it, so can I!

Up and Running is the perfect introduction to running. Yes, it's all about putting one foot in front of the other, but there's a proper way of doing it so you'll stay injury-free and fall in love with the sport.

Julia and Shauna's program is unique, as they give you a full eight weeks to complete it. This allows you to build a solid foundation of fitness and understand what it takes to be a runner. Unlike most programs, you'll be doing running drills right away that will teach you good technique and healthy habits. You'll be set up for a lifetime of running.

When people move too rapidly from couch to marathon they tend to drop out of the sport very quickly. Too much too soon is a recipe for injury and frustration. You'll enjoy your running more if you're patient and allow yourself to savour those gradual gains. This progressive program will help you do exactly that, and in the long run you'll be faster, stronger, and cover more distance.

Running isn't about how far you run, it's about how far you've come. Right now a mile may feel like a long way, but one day you'll look back and it will be merely a warm up.

My philosophy is, "never limit where running can take you." I mean that physically, emotionally, spiritually, and geographically. It's a powerful sport. I'm excited for you to begin your own running story. Let the eight weeks begin…

Bart Yasso
Chief Running Officer
Runner's World

Introduction
The Up and Running Plan

Running is a secret superpower. Whether it's chasing down your child in a supermarket, making a frantic dash for the bus, or running a **spontaneous** 5k race, being able to run is a portal to mind and body alignment.

It's not only **fantastic** for your fitness and quality of life, it's also a great source of community and connection. Running is an affordable and time-efficient workout that's easy to fit into our busy lives. It's a **foundation** for any sport or activity.

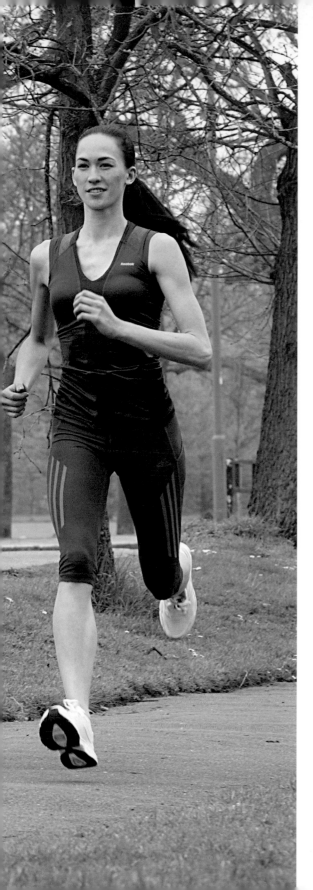

Running is also plain fun. It reconnects you to the joy of movement that we felt as kids. And it's never been easier to dive in and become a part of the vast running community. In the last few years, there's been a boom in accessible and entertaining 5k races—zombie runs, mud runs, and charity runs for all ages and levels.

This book will help you find your running superpowers. All you need to do is give us eight weeks, show up—and run.

Why This Plan Rocks

Most beginners' training plans are made up of simple run/walk segments. Other than running the risk of dying from boredom before finishing, many people struggle with this method as it's not adaptable to different fitness levels. Our plan meets you where you are, whether you've been inactive or involved in other types of exercise. We'll start conditioning your whole body for running from Day 1. The training plans are written in progressive sequence with powerful running drills incorporated into each week. At the end of Week 8 you'll be confident to run your first 5k.

Running is a mental exercise as much as a physical one. We'll set you up for success by helping you zoom in on your motivations, create achievable goals, and learn how to make running an integral and fulfilling part of your life.

Our Story

Shauna Reid had dreamed of being a runner but didn't think she ever could be one. In her mind, you had to be born a runner, like those guys with skinny legs and sweatbands pounding the streets at sunrise, or those chicks with the bouncing ponytails who glided on the treadmills at the gym.

Running wasn't for people like her—consistently bringing up the rear in the 100-meter dash at school, always picked last for softball, and unable to go more than 50 meters without coughing up a lung. As soon she graduated and was no longer forced to run, she gave up on the idea completely.

But then she met Julia Jones.

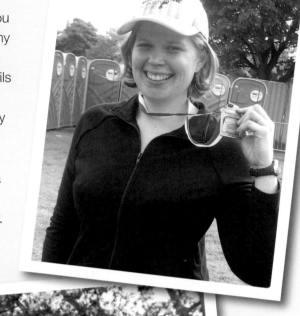

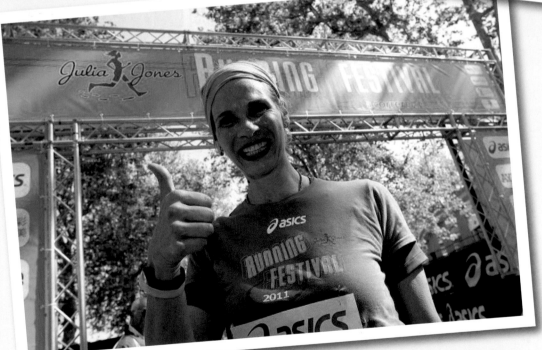

Top: Shauna Reid   Below: Julia Jones

Shauna had written about her impossible running dream on her blog. Julia had been a reader since Shauna moved from Australia to Scotland, and she felt a connection with her as she, too, was an expat, an American in Italy. She e-mailed Shauna to say that she was an expert running coach and would love to train her to run a 5k.

"No way," Shauna wrote back, "I can't run!"

But Julia said she had an amazing plan that had worked for thousands of people in her running clinics across Italy and she knew it would work for Shauna, too.

The fear in Shauna's stomach was outweighed by a kernel of excitement… What if Julia was right?

And so began eight weeks of hard work, lengthy e-mails, and amazing self-discoveries. Yes, there were tears. There were tantrums. There was that one time when Shauna's father-in-law asked whether she needed an ambulance, her post-run face was so red.

But the plan worked. It was fun. She loved ticking off each workout on her eight-week chart. She loved the fresh air on her face and her more defined calf muscles. And most of all, she loved those brief, thrilling moments when her legs seemed to float and she felt like…a runner.

When she finally crossed the line at her 5k race, she realized that Julia had been right about running. And she discovered that there was no greater feeling than taking your mind and body to a place you thought they couldn't go, a place you thought they didn't belong.

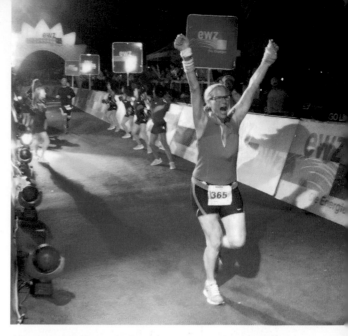

Julia Jones finishing at the Ironman race

This book will help you discover that feeling, too. Since Julia and Shauna's fateful meeting, that very same 5k training plan has helped thousands more people discover that they can be runners, via their wildly popular Up & Running online courses.

In this book they have refined and expanded the original training plan, adding all the wisdom they have gleaned from their runners. First, their eight-week program will take you from zero to 5k; then they give you a series of "Beyond the 5k Plans" to get you running even faster and stronger.

They have identified potential challenges and barriers, discovered the best strategies for keeping you motivated, and nailed down THE formula for running success. Together, they have the wisdom, the know-how, and the killer training plan to take you to your first 5k… and beyond.

So let's get started!

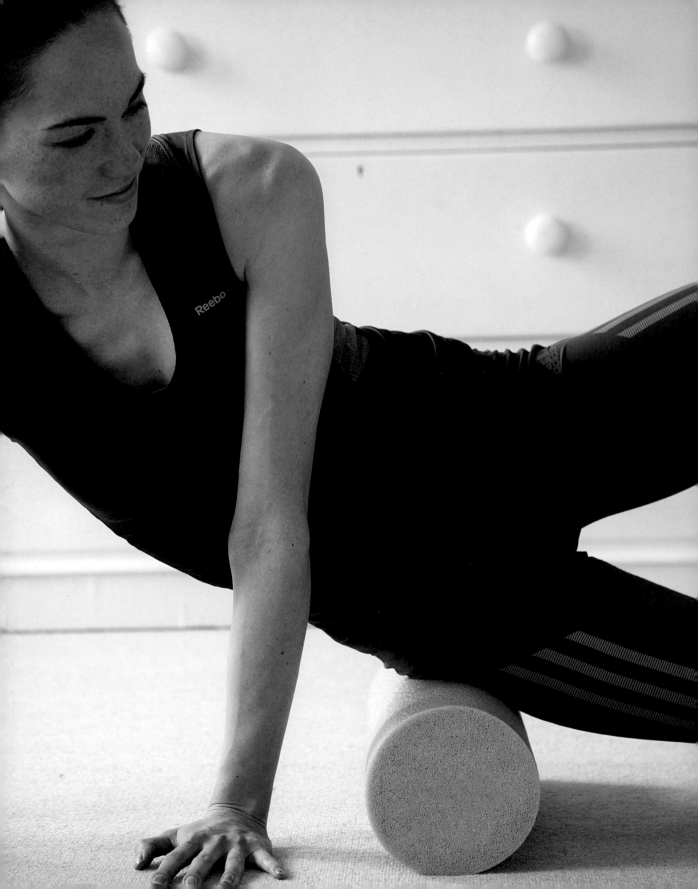

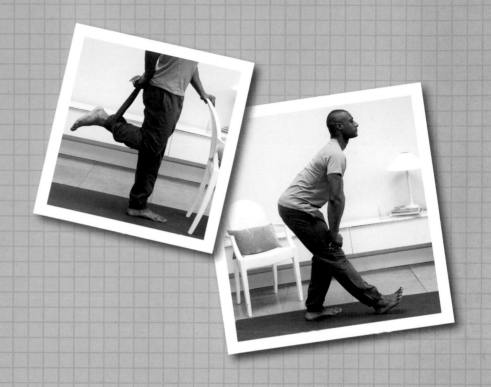

Warm-Up Week

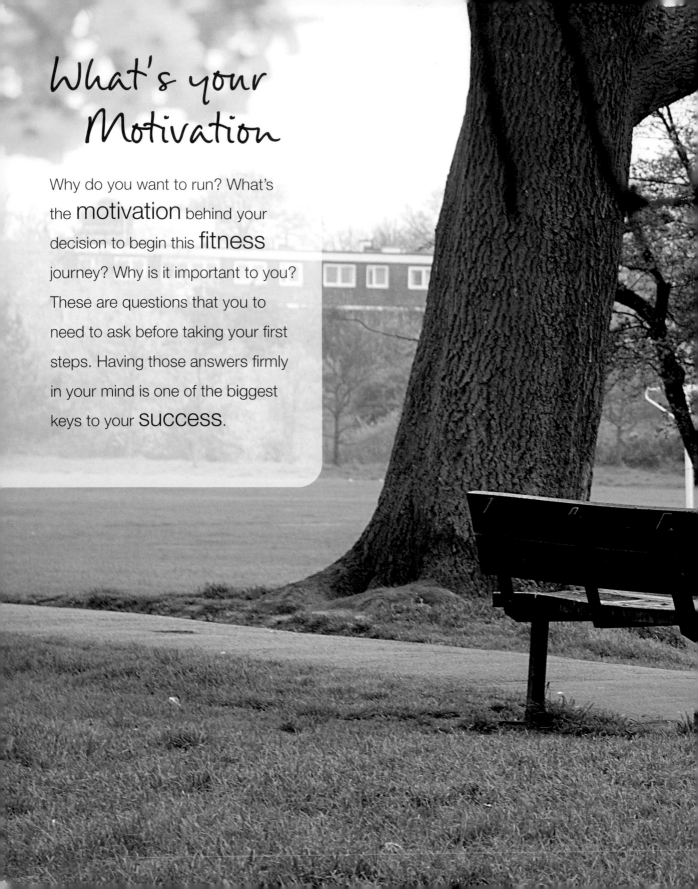

What's your Motivation

Why do you want to run? What's the **motivation** behind your decision to begin this **fitness** journey? Why is it important to you? These are questions that you to need to ask before taking your first steps. Having those answers firmly in your mind is one of the biggest keys to your **success**.

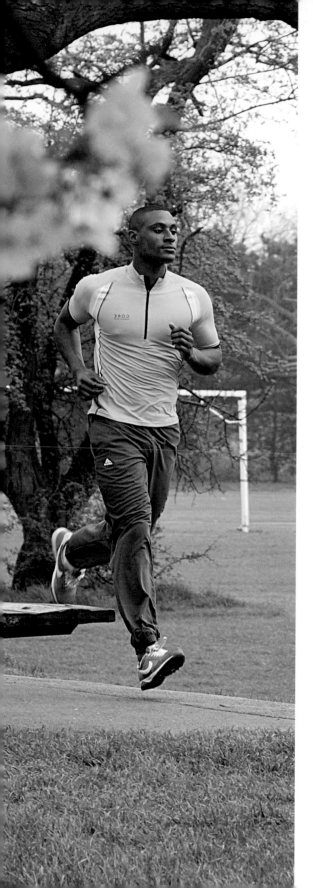

If you've ever watched children playing in a park or during a school recess, you'll notice that most of them share a habit: they don't walk, they run. They run from the swing to the slide. With a ball in hand, they run to the playing field. Sometimes they stop to examine a stick on the ground or chat with a playmate, then trot off at a quick clip to the next activity. The craziest ones to watch are children just let out from school. They topple over one another in their eagerness to dash out through the classroom door, bursting with pent-up energy and a desperate urge to move after so many hours of sitting still.

Some of us hang onto this energy well into our teens, pouring it into school athletics. But some of us outgrow the running habit right after elementary school as our bodies grow and transform every waking minute.

We become self-conscious about our changing bodies. Spontaneous movement is replaced by structured PE classes. What used to be fun is now an obligation. School sports are often more about competition rather than participation. If you're not good enough to make the team, there aren't as many opportunities to take part in sports. Unless you're a naturally athletic person or have a special talent, you will probably not be the first in line to try out for the volleyball team.

So for some of us, there's a pause. It can last a year or two—or five or twenty. With work, family, and community hogging our time, our energy reserves run low at the end of the day. Then out of the blue an idea pops up: "I want to run."

Perhaps you saw someone running in the park. They looked fit and happy and you want to be like that, too. You were shopping downtown and the road was blocked off for a local 5k charity race. You watched from behind the barriers and felt inspired by the huge variety of participants, thinking, "Maybe, just maybe, I could be running next year..."

Whatever your reason, there's a secret to being successful: your personal motivation.

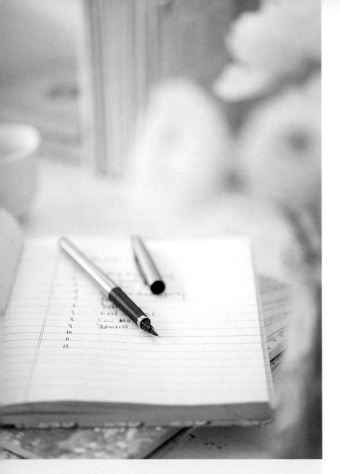

Task

Make a List of Your Motivations

Display them prominently where you can see them every day—it could be on your desk at work or on your refrigerator or kitchen cabinet at home. Write them on your bathroom mirror or turn them into a framed picture for an elegant reminder. Send yourself a daily e-mail, a phone reminder, or simply write them out in your diary. These visual reminders will help reinforce your motivation.

Why Run?

Knowing exactly what's behind your desire to run is the single most important component to completing this (or any) eight-week running program. Ask yourself: "Why am I doing this?"

You may be itching to skip ahead and get on with the training, but we urge you to stay with us. The truth is that despite the fantastic workout plans, training techniques, and expert advice in this book, following the plan is near impossible if you don't know why you're here.

Knowing your motivations will be what gets you lacing up your running shoes three days a week for the next eight weeks. It's easy to imagine your running adventure while you're reading a book, but when it's cold outside or you've had a bad day at work and just want to chill out on the couch, you'll need a compelling reason to get out the door. When the going gets tough, you can call upon these reasons to refuel your desire to keep going.

Strong motivations are usually accompanied by butterflies in your stomach or a tingly feeling in your chest whenever you think of that reason. It could be remembering your childhood love of running, the fear or thrill you felt when signing up for a race online, or picturing how you'll feel as you cross the finish line. You're pushing yourself out of your comfort zone—it's scary but you know it's the right thing to do. There's emotion involved, whether it's happiness or excitement or even anger.

Yes, there may be some negative emotions lurking behind your running urge. Maybe someone told you that you weren't made for running and you want to prove that person wrong. You're tired of feeling out of shape and saying, "I'll start over on Monday." Your sister or best buddy has embarked on a fitness kick and you envy their irritating enthusiasm. It's okay to be motivated by these feelings; just be sure to turn them into positive action.

Choose a Tangible Goal

A tangible goal is the perfect partner for your motivations. Tangible goals are essential for running as they help clarify where you are right now. They set a baseline and help you define what to do and the tools you need in order to get there.

What makes a goal tangible? It's measurable, specific, achievable, and helps you to focus your efforts. A lot of clients tell us, "Oh, I just want to run to get healthy." Running can help you get healthy, but you have to define "healthy" first.

We prefer to choose number-based goals, as numbers are concrete and measurable. They tell you how far away your goal is and how much more work you have yet to do. Based on the numbers, you'll easily know when you've achieved it.

You may have already achieved tangible goals in other areas of your life: going after a university degree, setting a savings target for a car or house deposit, challenging yourself to watch an entire "Mad Men" box set in one weekend.

Tangible goals also help create personal motivation. We all have a super secret goal that we haven't shared with anyone. Once you define that goal, you have a much better chance of obtaining it. And if you declare it to a friend? Practically done!

Task

Choosing a Tangible Running Goal

Here are a few ideas:

- **Complete the 24 workouts of the eight-week program.** Three workouts per week for eight weeks make 24 workouts. They do not need to be perfect workouts; you don't have to become Olympic material. Simply do each workout and you've achieved your goal. We've got some great visual ideas for counting down your workouts in the next section.

- **Time your 1km intervals.** From the very first week, you'll be doing timed 1km intervals. Write down your times each week and you'll start to see progress as you complete more and more workouts.

- **Track your cumulative mileage.** You could add up how many kilometers you cover in each workout and tally them up on a spreadsheet. Maybe you could bust out a fancy graph, too? Watching those numbers add up each week can be so motivating.

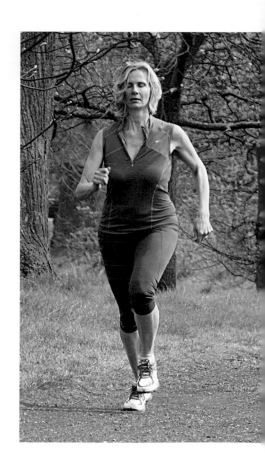

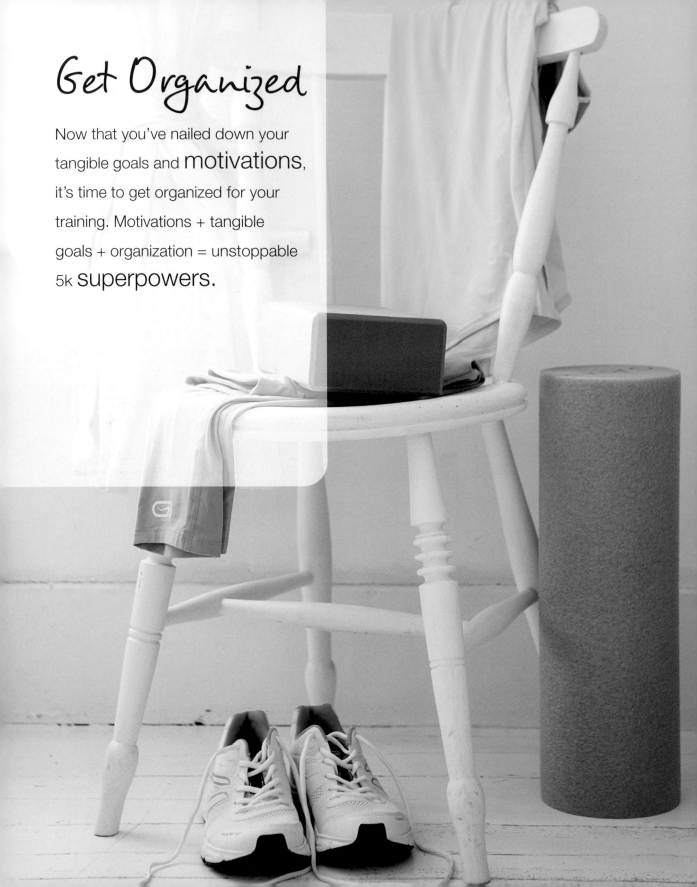

Get Organized

Now that you've nailed down your tangible goals and **motivations**, it's time to get organized for your training. Motivations + tangible goals + organization = unstoppable 5k **superpowers.**

Schedule your Workouts

You'll be running three times a week for the next eight weeks. Each session is approximately 40–50 minutes long. Get out your diary or calendar and schedule your three Week 1 workouts, allowing a rest day in between each session. Write it down in pen, not pencil, to seal your commitment. This is sacred, non-negotiable time; an un-missable hot date with yourself.

Choose your 5k Race

This is the pot of gold at the end of your eight-week training rainbow. Look for a 5k event for the weekend of your eighth week of training.

- The best race finders are online—Runners World and active.com have comprehensive listings.
- Find your nearest Parkrun—a free, timed, weekly 5k held in parks in nine countries, including the US, UK, Ireland, and Australia. With a friendly and inclusive atmosphere, they're perfect for a 5k debut.
- Run for a good cause and sign up for a Race for the Cure 5k event in the US or Race for Life in the UK.
- Check your local running store—they'll have flyers for local events.
- Don't worry if you can't find a 5k race in your area— you can create your own virtual event. Choose a date, then map out a route in your neighborhood or in a park; MapMyRun.com has a great route planner. Make it a day to remember by enlisting supportive friends and family to cheer you to the finish line. You could even make your own medal (large chocolate coins are ideal).

Once you've chosen your race, add it to your calendar and start dreaming of that finish line.

Decide How to Record your Progress

A training diary is an essential tool for tracking your progress and helping you see how far you've come. As well as recording the time and distance you run, you can record your thoughts about each workout, the weather, your mood, or anything else you want to note down. Trust us, you'll want to keep track of this stuff. Record your workouts in any way that suits your style. You could use any of these:

- The training diary worksheets on pages 156–157
- A running smartphone app, such as Runkeeper, to track mileage and generate fancy maps of your runs
- A paper diary
- An Excel spreadsheet

Create a Countdown

Think of a cool, visual way to count down your workouts and help you see your progress toward the 5k prize. Here are some ideas:

- Number some Post-it notes from 1–24, stick them on a wall, then rip one off after each workout.
- Make a paperclip chain and remove one after each workout.
- Draw a big red X on a calendar after each completed workout and be determined not to break the string of Xs.
- Put a dollar into a jar every time you finish a workout with the intention of treating yourself to a gift when you finish the course.

Gather your Gear

You don't need to go crazy buying lots of gear to get started. The bare minimum you need is:

- A good pair of running shoes
- Comfortable clothing
- For women, a supportive sports bra
- A simple sports watch or app, so you can time your runs

See the following pages for more detail and recommendations.

Gear Guide

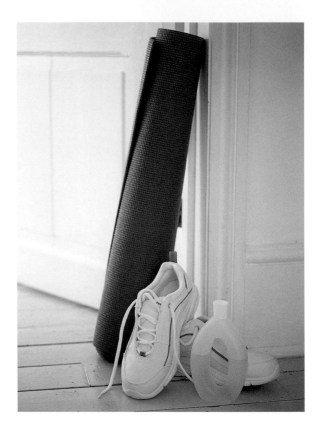

Shoes

Running shoes are the most important part of your running kit. Those ratty old sneakers lurking in the back of the wardrobe will not do. Your footwear is all that's protecting your body from the impact of your feet hitting the road. So treat yourself to a pair of well-fitted, quality running shoes that suit your feet.

Shopping for running shoes can be overwhelming, with all the jargon and wacky models on offer. We strongly recommend going to a specialist running store for your first purchase. It will save you time and money. You will often find the assistants are runners, experienced in fitting people of all ages, shapes, and sizes. They'll know what to look for and what models may suit you. Don't feel intimidated—you're a real runner and the staff are there to help.

Two Key Factors When Trying On Shoes

1 The biomechanics of your feet

We all have a natural way of running, our own personal style. If someone were to film you from behind while you ran, you'd notice that your running style would fall into one of the following categories:

Neutral

You're a neutral pronator; your foot naturally rolls inward upon landing while running. A small degree of pronation is natural.

Overpronation

Overpronation (or hyperpronation) occurs when the arch flattens out, thus stretching ligaments, tendons, and muscles. In all of Julia's years of coaching, she has seen very few true overpronators. Be careful of salespeople trying to convince you that you're an overpronator when in reality you just have naturally occurring pronation.

Underpronation (Supination)

You're an underpronator or supinator when your foot naturally rolls outward upon landing while running.

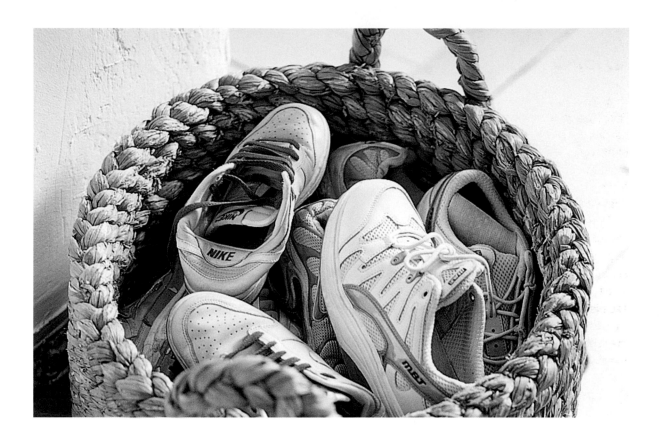

2 How often, how far?

The salesperson may ask how you'll be using the shoes—how often and how far will you be running? Let them know that you're just starting your running career and that you'll be training three times a week, with each workout taking you under an hour to complete.

When searching for your dream pair of running shoes, here are two things to look out for:

■ Make sure you have enough wiggle room in the toe-box area

As you run, your foot can move forward slightly inside your shoe. If you don't have a little room, you can say goodbye to a few of those toenails (ouch!). On the other hand, don't get your shoes too big or you'll end up with blisters from the friction of your foot sliding back and forth.

■ They must be comfortable right away

Make like Cinderella and keep trying different models until you find the one that fits your foot. We all have a different foot structure: wide, narrow, different length toes, high arches, no arches—the list goes on. Try on at least three or four pairs. Go for a test jog around the store. Some stores may have a treadmill just for the purpose. We promise that when you find the right pair, you'll know immediately.

In order to save a little cash, you can order your shoes online but you must go try them on first. Running shoes and sports shoes in general tend to run smaller than street shoes, so don't worry if you're a size and a half bigger than usual.

Socks

When you purchase your running shoes, throw in a few pairs of running or sports socks. They're made from a sweat-absorbing material without visible seams. They will keep your feet dry and help prevent blisters. They range from lightweight to heavily padded, so try a few pairs to see which you find most comfortable. They cost slightly more than regular socks, but if you only use them for running, they'll last longer.

Running Clothes

You don't need to rush out and buy fancy running clothes. There's no "right" way to dress, but it's essential that you wear something that feels comfortable while you're moving. What you wear also depends on the season and your local climate.

If you start to get more serious about running, you can invest in some technical running clothes. Unlike cotton clothing, synthetic fabrics such as CoolMax or Dri-Fit wick moisture away from your skin. Although the technical fabric running clothes may cost a little more, you'll appreciate the comfort, especially during longer runs. It can be motivating to invest in some running clothes—well-fitting running tights and a wicking top can make you feel the part more than baggy cotton trousers and an old T-shirt.

Essential for Women:
A Good Sports Bra

No matter what cup size you wear, you should always wear a sports bra for running. It will support your breasts and minimize movement. Sports bras also prevent any irritation that can be caused by fabric rubbing against your nipples, shoulders, and back. Since they're made from microfiber material, they'll absorb the sweat off your skin and keep you more comfortable.

In general, there are two models for sports bras: compression and regular closure bras. Most women opt for the compression bra as it's easy to slip on and off and everything stays in place. If you're well endowed you may want to try on a front-closure bra. They're designed for D cups and up.

Sports Watch

You'll need a simple sports watch to time your workouts. It doesn't need to be fancy, but it must have a chronograph that records your times. Another nice feature to have is laps, so that you can record the various intervals or sections of your workout.

Smartphone Apps

If you don't want to shell out for a sports watch, a smartphone app is a great alternative for keeping track of your workouts. If you've already forked out for the phone, the apps are relatively inexpensive and are packed with features such as lap count, calorie tracking, and route mapping. Some apps let you create your own workouts, so you can program the Up & Running training plans and have a bossy digital voice tell you what to do. However, these apps do tend to suck the life out of your battery, especially if you have the GPS enabled, so remember to charge your phone fully before you head out. Try Runkeeper, Runmeter, MapMyRun or Nike+ Running.

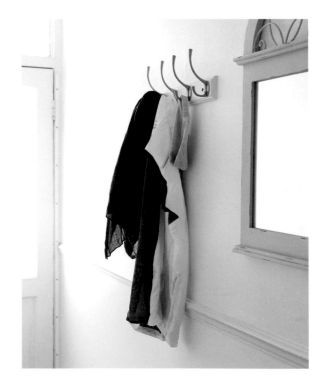

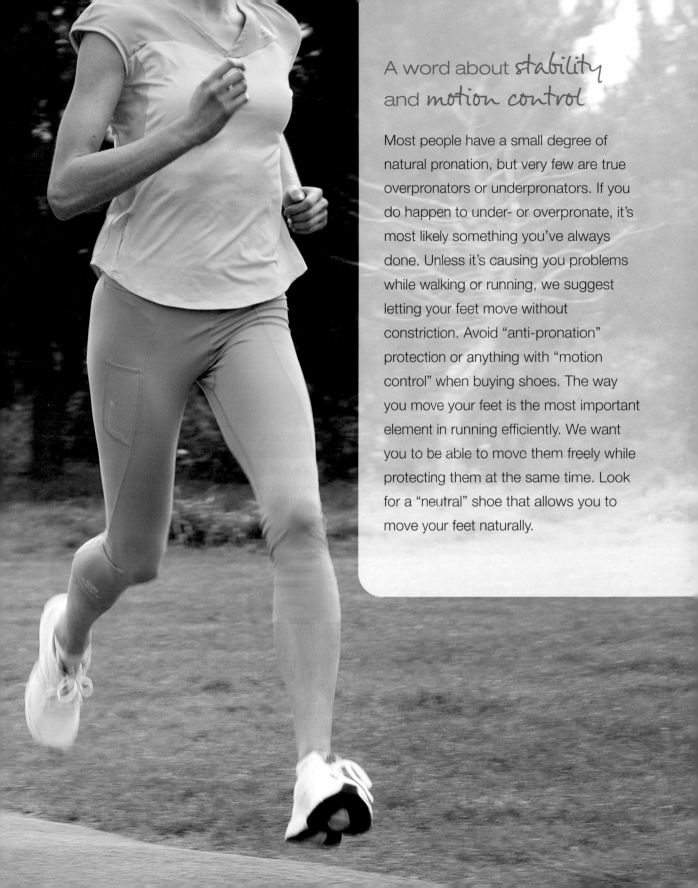

A word about *stability* and *motion control*

Most people have a small degree of natural pronation, but very few are true overpronators or underpronators. If you do happen to under- or overpronate, it's most likely something you've always done. Unless it's causing you problems while walking or running, we suggest letting your feet move without constriction. Avoid "anti-pronation" protection or anything with "motion control" when buying shoes. The way you move your feet is the most important element in running efficiently. We want you to be able to move them freely while protecting them at the same time. Look for a "neutral" shoe that allows you to move your feet naturally.

Running Routes

You don't need a lot of space to start your running adventure. Sure, a wide country road without traffic would be ideal, along with clear blue skies and birds singing from the trees. But don't be discouraged if that's not what's waiting outside your front door. Look around and see where other runners are working out. Most communities have a running "Mecca" where everyone seems to congregate.

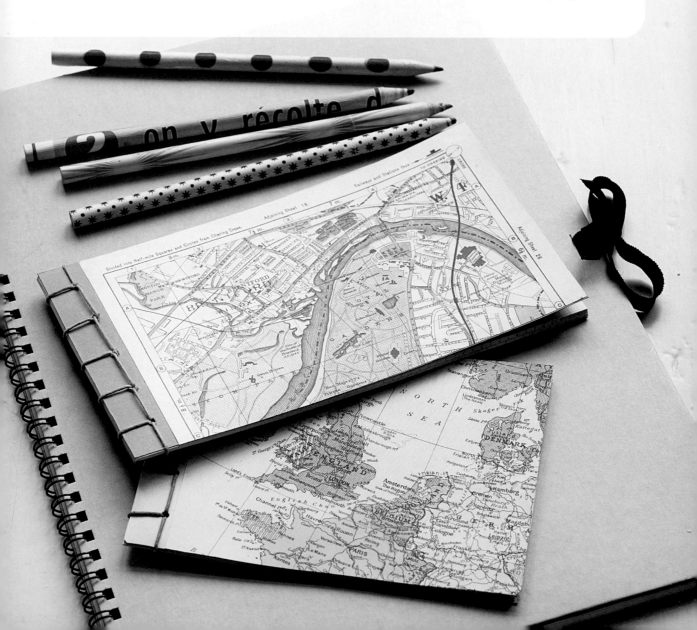

Yes to:

- Parks are one of the best places to run. They can have running paths, trails, or outdoor gym equipment to complement your workout. But the best reason to run in a park is the natural environment that surrounds you. Trees, bushes, and shrubs help filter some of the air polluted by nearby traffic.

- Bike paths are ideal for running as they're closed to car traffic. You can run for quite a long distance without any worries. You do need to be careful of the cyclists, though. Just stay to the side of the path and keep your eyes and ears open for bike traffic.

- Athletic tracks are popular with beginners—they're safe, with no cars or crazy fast cyclists to worry about. Most have a warm-up circuit that encompasses the track, sometimes on the other side of a fence. You could do your own warm-up there or use it for a change of scenery during your workout. If there are other athletes using the track, remember the number one rule: the fastest runners occupy the first lane. Use it if you need to time your 1k, but otherwise walk or run on the perimeter of the oval.

Be careful with:

- Footpaths are typically made of concrete, which is a mix of cement and sand or gravel. It's hard and durable, but also hard on your body if you're running on it. Footpaths are often poorly maintained, so when cracks or crevices appear, they stay forever, or at least until the city council gets enough complaints to fix them. Uneven surfaces can be quite dangerous for inexperienced runners with unsteady gaits and weak ankles. If you need to use a footpath to get to a park to run, try a fast walk for your warm-up instead.

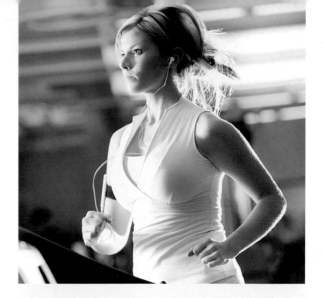

We understand that sometimes outdoor running isn't possible. In those cases, doing a workout on a treadmill is better than no workout at all. We've included a treadmill option in each week's workout. Try to think of the treadmill as a last-resort option and not a regular practice—remember that those fun 5k races are all going to be on the road.

- Beaches—can you see yourself running on the sand at sunset just like in "Chariots of Fire" with the Vangelis music theme swelling in the background? Well, put that fantasy on hold for now because running on sand is one of the most difficult exercises. It's great for muscle strengthening and raising anaerobic threshold, but we recommend that you wait until you've been running for a while.

- Running outdoors and running on a treadmill are two quite different activities. Running on a treadmill might feel easier, because it actually is. First of all, you're indoors, so there's no wind resistance. The machine also does some of the work for you since there is a mechanical belt rolling beneath your feet and you don't actually have to use your own force (hamstrings and glutes) to propel yourself forward.

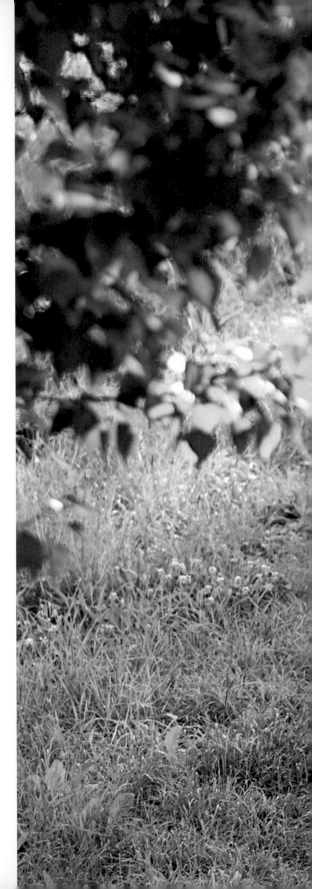

About the Training Plan

The Up & Running 5k program is an eight-week schedule with three workouts per week. It's essential that you follow the plans exactly as written. You must run three times per week, no more and no less. Don't alter or reorder the plans. They are planned out in a progressive sequence to increase your fitness gradually while avoiding injury.

Each workout lasts around 40–50 minutes. Don't worry if you take more or less time than this. It all depends on your current fitness level, and the beauty of the plan is that it works with where you are right now.

The workouts are broken down into three parts:

1. **The warm-up**
2. **Exercises or drills**
3. **Longer running segments**

Free Form Running

You'll see the term "Free Form Running" in each workout. It simply means that you can cover the given distance in whatever way you feel comfortable in that moment. It could mean:

- Walking
- Walking at a brisk pace
- Alternating between walking and running
- Begin walking and end with running
- Running at a slow pace
- Beginning at a slow pace and then running progressively faster
- Plain old running

Don't worry about whether you are doing it "right." There is no right or wrong here! Relax, enjoy yourself, and listen to your body. Just don't underestimate how much you're capable of doing. Be consistent and your Free Form Running will transform into something you enjoy, however you happen to interpret it.

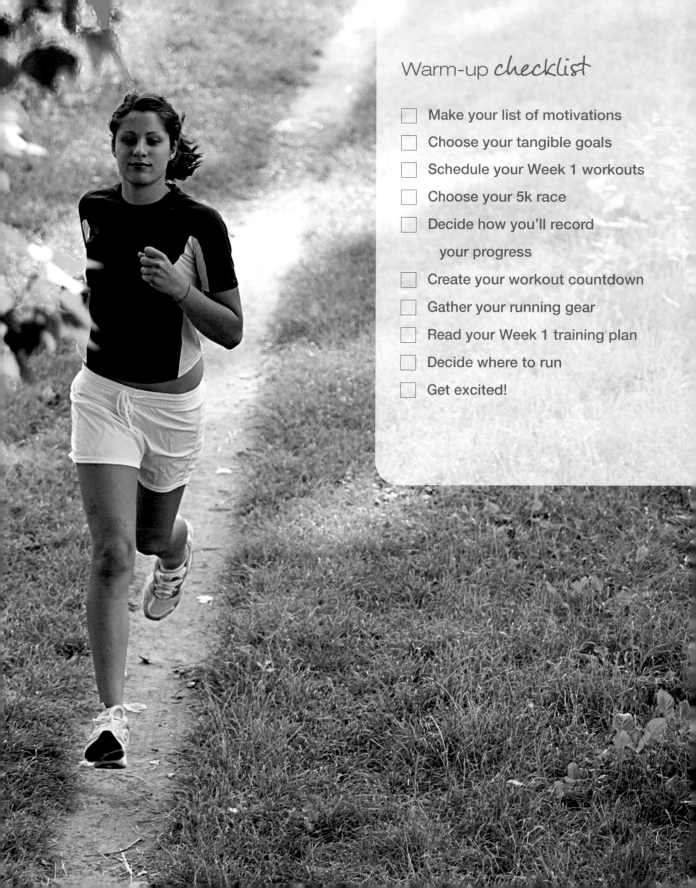

Warm-up *checklist*

- [ ] Make your list of motivations
- [ ] Choose your tangible goals
- [ ] Schedule your Week 1 workouts
- [ ] Choose your 5k race
- [ ] Decide how you'll record
     your progress
- [ ] Create your workout countdown
- [ ] Gather your running gear
- [ ] Read your Week 1 training plan
- [ ] Decide where to run
- [ ] Get excited!

Week 1 Exercise
Stretches

You'll find stretch breaks in your weekly training plans, right after the warm-up and again at the end of the workout. This is simply our recommendation—you don't have to do both stretch segments if you don't want to. Our only rule is that you should never stretch before you've warmed up.

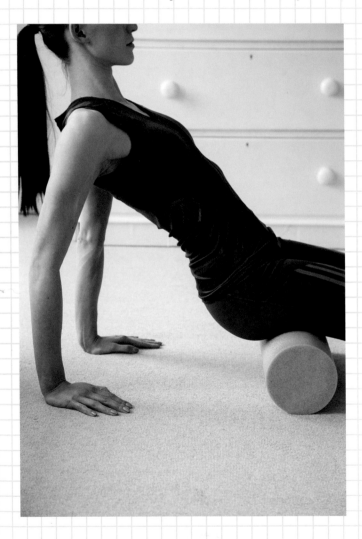

If you're already familiar with stretching, go ahead and spend those few minutes after the warm-up stretching out and/or walking around as you see fit. But if you'd like some guidance on how to stretch, our stretch sequence below hits all the major muscles in five simple moves.

While you stretch, keep in mind why you're doing it:

Stretching helps to elongate your muscles, thus giving you a greater range of motion.

Tight muscles can shorten your stride and/or change your posture, which can increase the risk of injury. A good range of movement is important for long-term injury prevention.

You don't need to become a super bendy yoga master. Just start from where you are and work on gradually increasing your flexibility.

Arm and Shoulder Stretch

TARGET MUSCLES: deltoids, scapula, and biceps

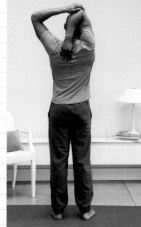
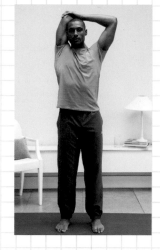

1 Stand with your feet approximately shoulder-width apart. Start with your right arm. Raise it straight up, then bend it at the elbow, placing your hand on your back.

2 Stay in position for 30 seconds and then repeat the exercise using your left arm.

Note that one side of your body will feel more flexible than the other. How far down you can place your hand will depend on your flexibility. It may be at the base of your neck or toward the middle of your back.

Calf Stretch

TARGET MUSCLE: gastrocnemius, i.e. calf muscle

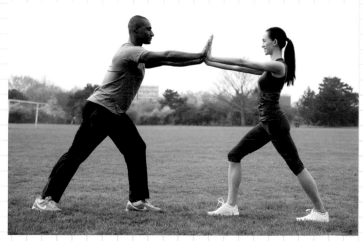
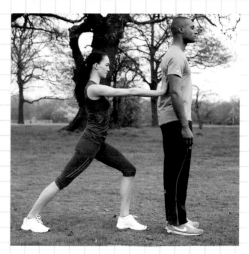

1 Place your right foot behind you. You can do this with your hands at your sides or on your hips. You could also brace your hands against a wall or another person, like in the photograph.

2 Lean forward and feel the gentle effect of the stretch in the extended leg. Hold your position for about 30 seconds. No bouncing! Then switch and stretch the opposite leg.

Quadricep Flex

TARGET MUSCLES: Quadriceps, inguinal ligament, i.e. the front of your thigh

1 Stand up straight. Lift your right foot behind you, holding your right foot with your right hand. Pull your foot slowly toward your glute. Feel your quadricep stretching.

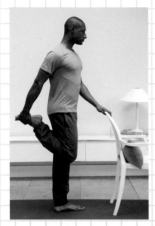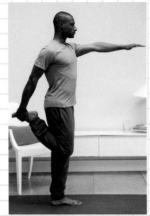

2 Keep your knees as closely together as possible. You can hold a hand out in front of you for balance if you need to. Hold the stretch for no longer than 30 seconds and then repeat with your left leg.

If you're having difficulty grabbing hold of your foot, try these options:

- Wear long pants and instead of grabbing your ankle, hold on to a piece of fabric from the hem.
- Use a rope or a towel to grab your ankle, then gently pull the rope or towel toward you. You can put your other hand on a wall or chair for balance.

Hamstring Stretch

TARGET MUSCLES: semitendinosus, semimembranosus, biceps femoris (collectively, the hamstring)

1 From a standing position, extend one leg in front of you. Plant the heel firmly on the ground with your toes pointing upward.

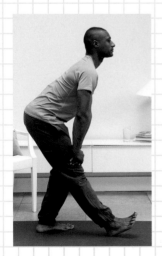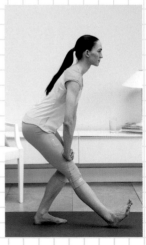

2 With your knees locked, slowly bend forward onto the extended leg. Stretch down as far as you comfortably can. You can place your hands on your thigh or knee if you like. When you feel you've arrived at your maximum extension, hold the pose for one minute. Breathe deeply while you hold the pose.

You may also feel this stretch in your back or calves, but the hamstring is your primary target.

Standing Forward Bend

TARGET MUSCLES: Lower back extensor muscles, hamstring muscles, abdominal muscles

There are several variations possible for this pose but for all options, start with your feet approximately shoulder-width apart, bend your knees slightly and bend down from your hips. Straighten your legs until your knees are no longer bent. Then relax your neck and shoulders. Depending on your flexibility, you can now:

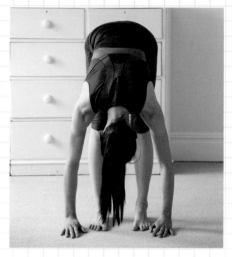

Place your palms on the floor.

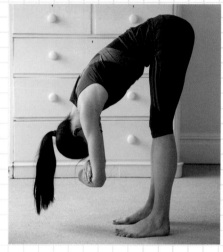

Cross your forearms, hold your elbows, and hang forward.

Simply hang forward with straight arms.

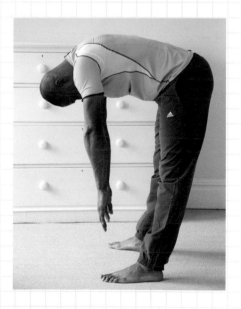

Stay in your chosen position for 30–60 seconds. Bend your knees and place your hands on your thighs as you come up to avoid placing strain on your back.

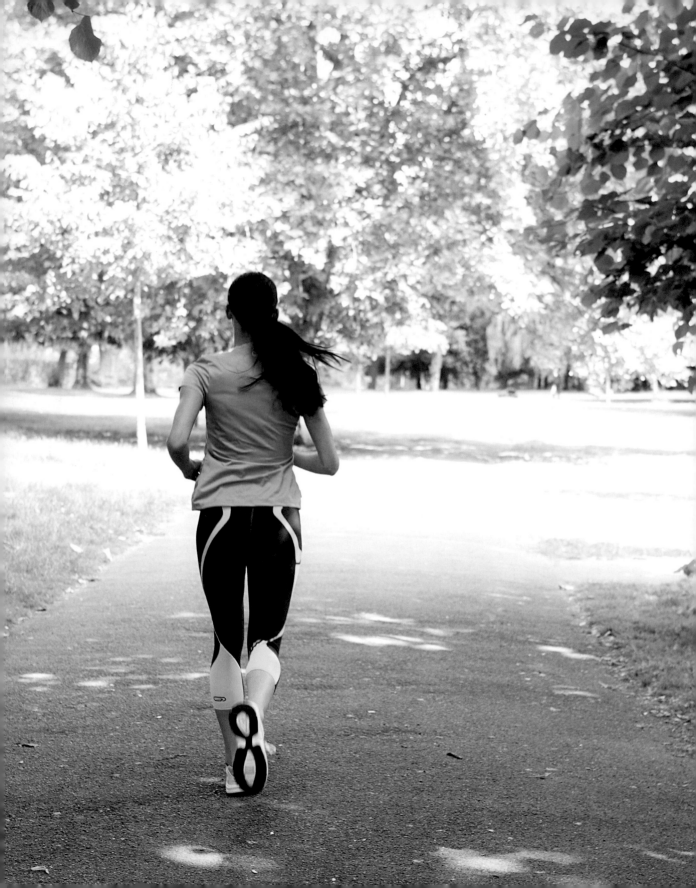

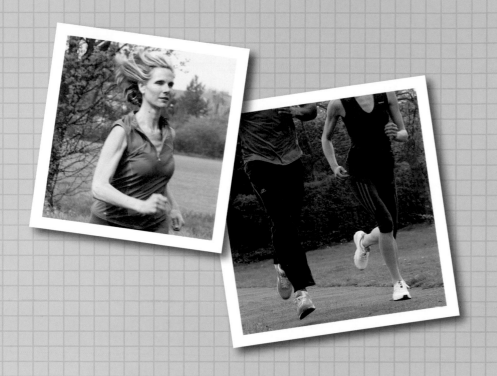

Making Time to Run

How to Make Time

We all have the same amount of time available to us. Twenty-four hours equal **1,440 minutes**, wherever you live in the world. How we **utilize** our time is what we need to look at. People often say to us, "I'd love to run, but I don't have as much **free time** as you do." Or, "I wish I had more time, but I just can't find any right now. Maybe someday!"

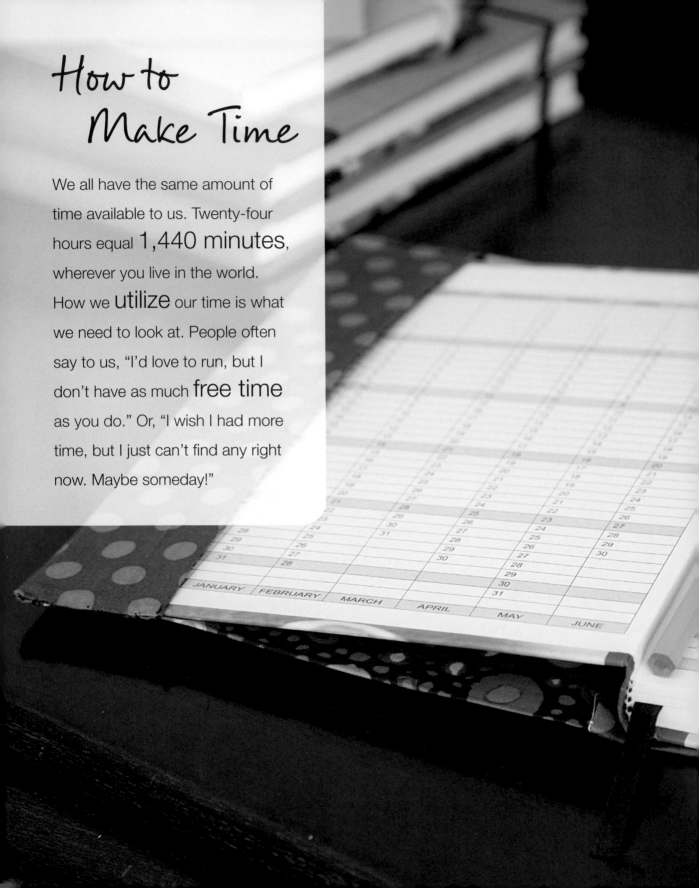

You may be working full time or part time or have a long commute. You may have children or pets or volunteer work. But if you really want to begin this running adventure, you need to examine your own 24 hours and plan for that time. We'll show you how it's done.

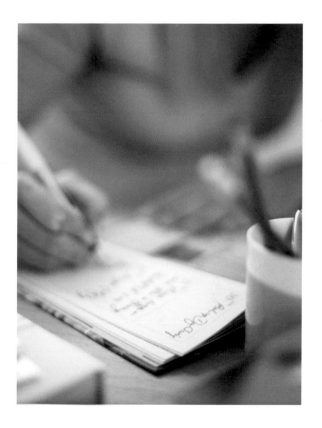

Make your Health a Priority

You're a wonderful caregiver with a to-do list growing faster than you can cross things off. You can't say no when you're asked to switch with a colleague for the late shift. You take on yet another volunteer committee at your children's school. Then it all comes to a screeching halt the minute you come down with a cold, fever, or worse.

You must make your health a priority. An easy way to rewire your thinking is to remember that good health is the foundation for everything that happens in life. It means taking care of yourself in every way possible, both physically and mentally.

Put yourself at the top of your own to-do list. Moving your body is an essential part of taking care of your health and not a selfish act. We'll talk more about this later in the chapter.

Block Off Essential Activities

Take out your diary and examine one week at a time. Block off your work hours and weekly appointments so that you can see your free time clearly.

Examine How you Spend your Time

There's always some mindless television watching and Internet surfing that can be reduced. Think about revamping some of your daily routines. Meals can be prepared ahead of time or, better yet, try new recipes with conservative cooking times. Outfits planned and laid out the night before can save minutes of frantic searching for something to wear in the morning.

Make your Running Time Non-Negotiable

That means it's a fixed appointment. When it's time for your scheduled workout, don't ask yourself if you "feel" like going or wonder whether maybe today's not the "right" day to run. Get dressed and go. You can ponder the merits of your run after it's done, perhaps while lounging in your robe and sipping a glass of sparkling water. Beforehand, it's just distraction and self-sabotage.

Getting Out the Door

Runners make it look so simple.
They bounce along with their
earphones plugged in, singing off-
key with a smirk on their faces.
They **jog** in place as they wait at
the traffic lights, as if they just can't
stop those **legs** from moving.
How do they do it?

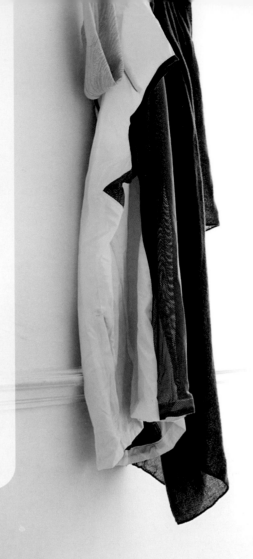

Why does getting out the door for a run feel like a monumental task to you? You push the snooze button one too many times. The phone rings and the conversation (deliberately?) eats up your workout time. You sit on the couch after work for just one moment, only to wake a few hours later and it's dark outside. You'll try again tomorrow. Promise!

Despite appearances, even seasoned runners can have a difficult time convincing themselves to lace up their shoes. They've just cultivated clever tactics to squash any resistance.

Here's how to make it easier:

- **Do your workout in the morning.** You'll have a much better chance of getting your run finished if you head out before anyone else is up, demanding your attention, and before work takes your head to another place. This usually works best if you're already an early riser, but if you're not, try a few morning runs—you may be surprised at how good it feels to be out and about while the rest of the world dozes on. Set the scene to make it more enticing: have your coffee ready to percolate or lay the breakfast table for when you return.

- **Lay out your clothes in advance.** You can waste a lot of time making sartorial decisions or searching for the perfect pair of running shorts. If your running clothes are set out ahead of time, there's no scope for procrastination. Once you're dressed and ready to run, you've won half the mental battle.

- **Avoid electronic distractions.** No checking your e-mail or announcing your run to your online friends—you'll inevitably disappear down the Internet rabbit hole. Leave social media until after your workout and post a triumphant sweaty selfie.

- **Connect with a positive feeling.** What do you love most about running? Maybe it's after the workout is done and you're taking a hot, steamy shower; or that

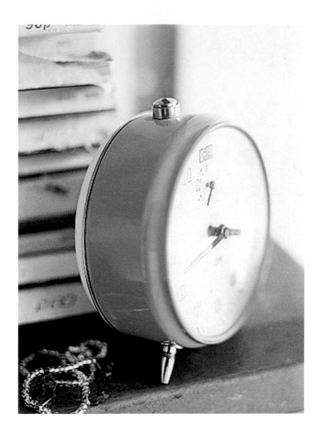

moment while you're running and realize, "Hey, I'm doing this!" Tap into what gets you excited about running and let it carry you out the door.

- **Make a running date with a friend.** You may let yourself down but we bet you'd never dream of doing that to a friend; especially if you're meeting in a park at the crack of dawn.

- **Do not ask questions.** While you're driving home from work don't ask yourself if you feel like running. Be robot-like: put on those running clothes and get out the door. We guarantee that after the first 10 minutes, you'll start to feel better, energized and in the mood to move. You may even get one of those running smirks on your face, too.

What motivates runners to get out the door?

It can be challenging to get into the habit of running regularly and it's important to think of ways to motivate yourself. We hope the runners' comments below will give you some ideas.

Rewarding myself. Don't underestimate the power of the sticker. ANG, AUSTRALIA

My brain is always trying to talk me out of running, so the best trick is not to pay any attention to it— it's just throwing a tantrum. As I put on my running clothes, it says, "I'm tired!" As I choose my music, it complains about my weary legs. It's still whining even as I open the door. But more action equals less talk, plus a greater chance of doing the run. And I feel oh-so-smug afterward.

PAULA, UNITED ARAB EMIRATES

The desire to escape from my wife.

MICHELE, ITALY

My pedometer helps with accountability. Knowing my online friends can see my step count is very motivating. NIKKI, USA

A new playlist. CLAUDIO, ITALY

Completing a workout makes me feel in control of my life, because I have achieved something. Each workout is a sign that I can succeed. Even if a run is my only accomplishment that day, whatever the distance, it's something I can hold on to. KAT, UK

It's the joy of being outside. With the British weather it would be so easy to stay indoors all the time. I love that I have an excuse to get out and see the seasons change.

PAULA, UK

Knowing how guilty I'd feel if I didn't go. ETTORE, ITALY

Week 1 superstar profile: Sara Lando

Age: 35
Location: Bassano del Grappa, Italy
Occupation: Photographer

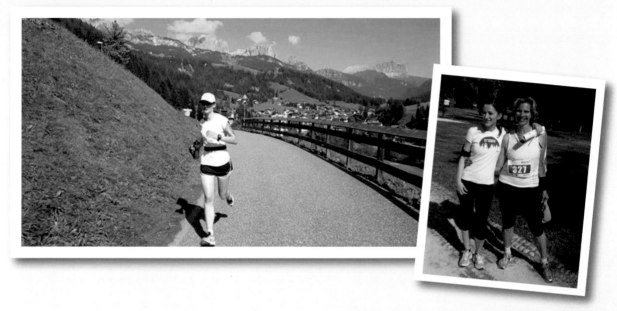

I was always bad at running. PE was the only subject I dreaded at school. But I secretly wished I could enjoy running because it sounded perfect for me: a solitary, repetitive activity in which I could get lost.

One day I was complaining about being lazy and stressed and a friend suggested I try running. But I just couldn't get past the "run four minutes" stage of the plan I was trying to follow.

Then I met Julia and fell in love with her practicality and no-BS attitude. The moment she launched Up & Running with Shauna, I did something crazy: I signed up.

Those first eight weeks were hard, amazing, intoxicating, and filled with awesomeness. Running my first 5k was exhilarating. Not only was I doing something I'd never thought I'd be able to do, but I was loving it. In the years since my first Up & Running 5k

course, I've worked my way up to a 10k, half marathon, and finally the mighty marathon.

The weirdest thing about running is that no matter how miserable I feel during a workout, I always feel good when I'm done.

Running made me realize that I'm stronger than I think. I've learned that I am not a quitter, and that surprised me.

My advice? Only worry about the workout you're about to do and ignore what's coming next week, because it'll always seem too much. But it won't be, because next week you'll be a different runner.

Enjoy the process. The final race is just the crowning of the whole thing, but you'll find out that the feeling of accomplishment at the end of some of those training runs is just as satisfying.

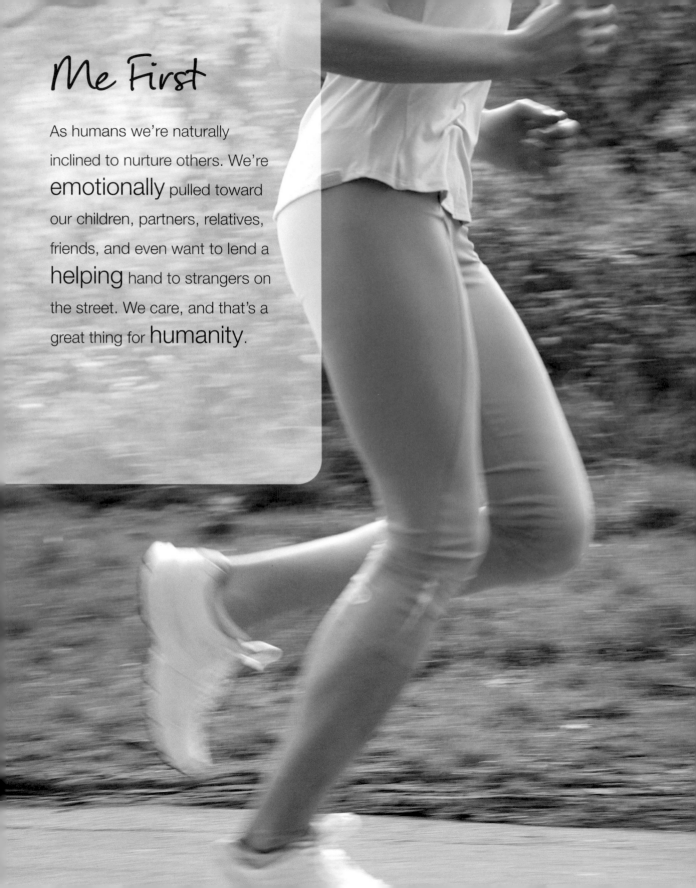

Me First

As humans we're naturally inclined to nurture others. We're **emotionally** pulled toward our children, partners, relatives, friends, and even want to lend a **helping** hand to strangers on the street. We care, and that's a great thing for **humanity**.

Some of us are born caregivers. It's these generous souls who have the most difficult time caring for themselves. Taking time for an exercise program or even to go for a walk seems like an insurmountable task. We've found this true especially when it comes to parents with small or special needs children. There's so much on their daily to do lists that the last person they consider is themselves. But not only do you deserve and need time for physical activity, it benefits your loved ones, too.

Think of your life activities as a big pyramid. The bottom layer consists of your family and work, often overlapping each other. As you build up to the top, there are daily meals to prepare, a house to maintain, and friends and relatives to interact with. Then, at the very top, there are a few social obligations.

So where does your health fit in the pyramid?

In reality, your health needs to be at the base, because that is what holds up the entire structure. If you care for yourself first, your pyramid will have a strong foundation. You'll feel more balanced and have more energy. It is not a selfish act. If you don't prioritize your health, the pyramid will slowly crumble. Physical activity is one of the key ingredients to feeling your best. You'll be able to give more and care more if you're coming from a healthy place, both in body and mind.

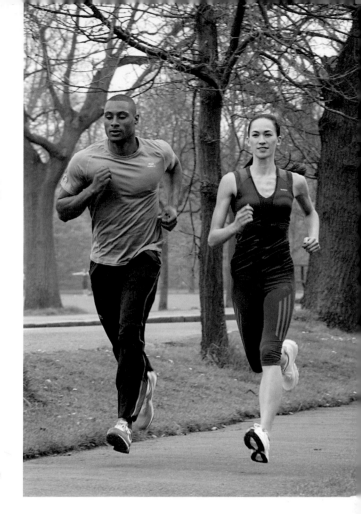

Don't Be Afraid to Ask for Support

In order to complete 24 workouts over the next eight weeks, you may need to do some life rearranging. This could involve asking for support. That may be a horrifying thought if you're one of those selfless caregivers who usually do things on their own. But asking for support isn't always about asking for people's time. It's more about letting your loved ones know that this project is important to you. It can be as easy as:

- Asking your partner gently to coax you out the door for your workout, no matter how reluctant you seem when the time comes
- Having your children ride their bikes beside you on your run
- Asking a colleague to reschedule a meeting so you can sneak in a lunchtime workout
- Asking a family member to keep an eye on the dinner while you're out
- Making a pact with friends to text after every run and asking them to chase you if you don't report in a timely manner

Week 1
Training Plan

- Brisk walk — 5:00
- Walk with arm swings — 3:00
- Stretch — 3:00
- 10 x (walk 0:30/slow run 0:10) — 6:40
- 1km walk
- 1km Free Form Run

Instructions

1 Brisk walk
Walk for five minutes at a brisk pace. This is a warm-up to get your blood circulating and body moving.

2 Walk with arm swings
Continue walking for another three minutes while swinging your arms intermittently. This is to get your circulation active through your shoulders and arms. Aim for 10 back and forth swings for every minute.

3 Stretch
Take three minutes to stop for a good stretch. Check out our stretch routine in the Warm-Up chapter. Stretching should always be done after your warm-up, or you can leave it until after you've completed the workout.

Stagger your workouts
Leave a day between each workout if possible. You can do other forms of exercise if you wish—just not running.

Take a break
If you need to rest a moment between steps, that's fine. You might want to take a minute or two to gather yourself between the two 1km intervals.

FAQ

Q. Do I need to take water on my workout?

A. The 5k workouts are short in duration so you probably won't need to take water with you. Remember that hydration is an all-day project—you need to be drinking water throughout the day as well as eating fresh, raw vegetables and fruit. That way, when workout time comes around, your body is well hydrated and ready to go. If it's an exceptionally hot day and you get a dry mouth when you run, put a few fluid ounces of water into a plastic bottle, scrunch it up, and carry it in your pocket.

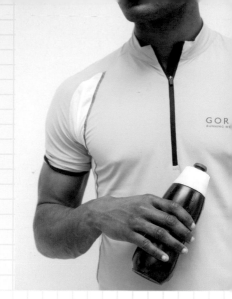

4 **10 x (walk 0:30/ slow run 0:10)**
This circuit has you alternating between walking and slow running. It should flow smoothly without any jerky movements. That's 30 seconds of brisk walking and 10 seconds of slow running, repeated 10 times (six minutes and 40 seconds in total).

5 **1km walk**
Walk at a fast pace and time it.

6 **1km Free Form Run**
Repeat the same distance. Run, walk, or Free Form Run— whatever feels right for you. The important thing is that you take less time than for the 1km walk. Write your times in your training diary later so you can chart your progress.

Be patient
If you're consistent, you should see progress right away. Consistency is everything!

Week 1 Wisdom
Everything was kind of wrong tonight. I was sore, it was getting dark, I was being bitten by mosquitoes, and I swallowed a bunch of midges. Yet for some reason the run felt good. Ah, running. Who can fathom thy mysteries?
JAMES, CANADA

Treadmill Modifications
- For the arm swings, choose a version that allows you to maintain your balance.
- Hop off the treadmill for the stretching.

Week 1 Exercise
Arm Swings

Your workout starts with a warm-up walk, adding in arm swings. The arm swings get the blood circulating and help relax your arms and shoulders. Arm swings can be done in any of the following ways:

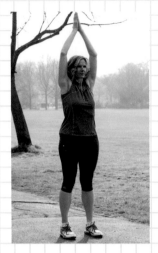

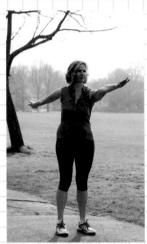

1 Stand with feet slightly apart and arms raised above your head.

2 Bring one arm forward as the other moves back.

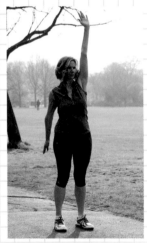

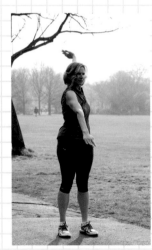

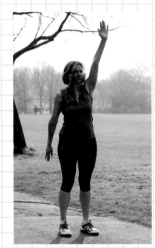

3 Continue rotating both arms so that the front arm points toward the sky and the back arm points at the ground.

4 Continue the rotation by bringing the back arm forward and moving the leading arm behind.

5 One rep is complete when you return to the starting position. Continue with the exercise, alternating both arms either backward or forward.

This exercise can be tiring if you're not used to using your shoulders, so don't overdo it. Aim for 10 back and forth swings per minute.

Variation 1

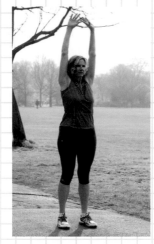 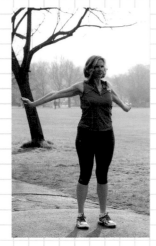 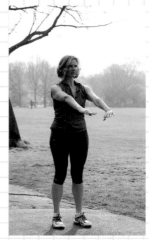

1 Stand with feet slightly apart and bring both arms up over your head.

2 Bring the arms backward.

3 And finish by bringing them forward.

Variation 2

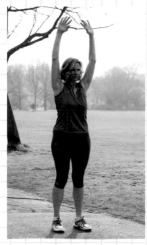 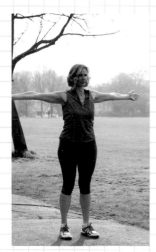 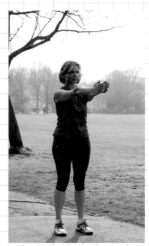

1 Raise your arms toward the sky and hold for five seconds.

2 Open your arms wide.

3 Clap your hands (gontly) in front of your chest.

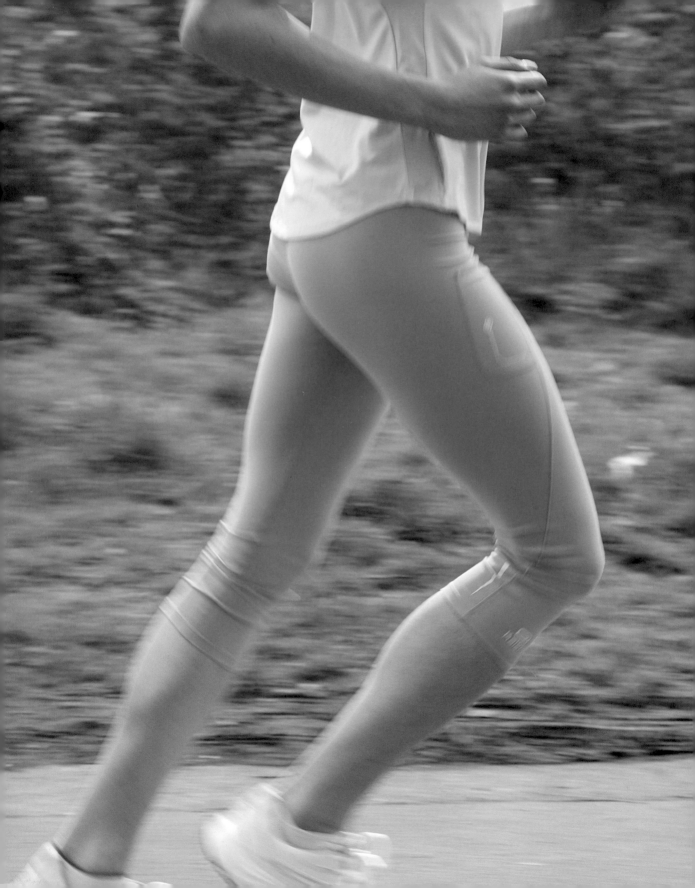

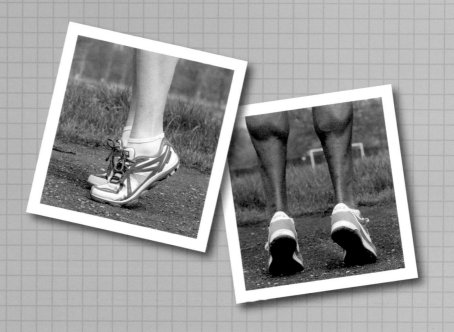

Your Body as a Well-Oiled Running Machine

You and your Feet

It's a gorgeous, sunny day and you decide to drive to the beach to enjoy the rays. You step onto the sand and what's the first thing you do? Most people, no matter their age, instantly take off their shoes. There's something so pleasurable about warm sand squeezing between your toes. The grains of sand mold themselves to your feet and you're transported back to happy childhood vacations.

Unfortunately, nowadays most of us spend every minute of the day in a pair of constricting shoes. At home we wear slippers. Outdoors we're in heavy boots, dress shoes, or even impossible four-inch heels. Yes, shoes are essential and fun; we're not downplaying that. But most of us rarely use our feet in the way they're meant to be used. Trapped inside shoes from morning to night, our feet rarely stretch out or touch a bare floor.

As a new runner, you may be thinking about improving your lung capacity or toning those quadriceps and glutes. We ask you instead to think about your feet. They're the two most important parts of a runner's body. How you use your feet will make or break your running career.

Consider your feet as functional. They're shaped to complement and support the body they're attached to—whether that be short, wide, long, or narrow. Each foot contains 28 bones, 33 joints, over 40 muscles and tendons, and about 100 ligaments. More than 25 percent of the bones in our body are concentrated in those two appendages.

Feet need training and conditioning just like rest of the body. The strength and agility of your feet directly influences:

- How efficiently you push off the ground as you run
- Your gait pattern
- Ankle stability
- Body balance

Unconditioned feet will lead to problems further up the kinetic chain, such as shin fatigue, knee pain, hip and back aches.

When you run, you instinctively use whatever part of your body is the strongest—you don't have much control over that. Most beginners (and some with quite a few miles logged) exclusively use their quadriceps, landing on unconditioned feet and pushing off from their knees. This style of running not only does damage to your body, it also requires a lot of energy. The secret to dynamic, injury-free running is to have supple, reactive feet.

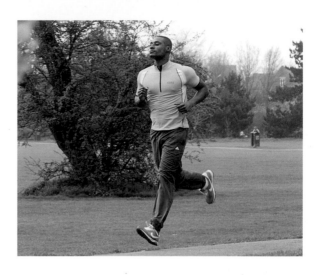

Work your Feet
You'll be doing all sorts of foot agility drills in your 5k training. They may sound crazy at first, but skipping, heel lifts, and doing "The Stork" are all designed to reactivate dormant foot muscles and ligaments. You can also help your feet by massaging them for a few minutes in the evening with calendula oil, a natural anti-inflammatory that helps to soothe sore muscles.

Go Barefoot at Home
Slip on a pair of socks if your toes get cold. Simply walking around your house without shoes will get you using your feet in a different way and help compensate for all the hours they spend trapped in leather.

Be Aware of your Feet as You Run
Try placing your attention on your feet for just 30 seconds during a workout. Feel where your feet land. Is it on the heel or the mid-sole? Do you naturally push yourself forward or do you shuffle? Listen to the sound of your footsteps. Is there a steady pitter-patter or a scraping sound? Don't try to modify anything at this stage, just start to be aware of what your feet are doing. Once you've been running for a good month, we'll start to look at your running style.

The Stork

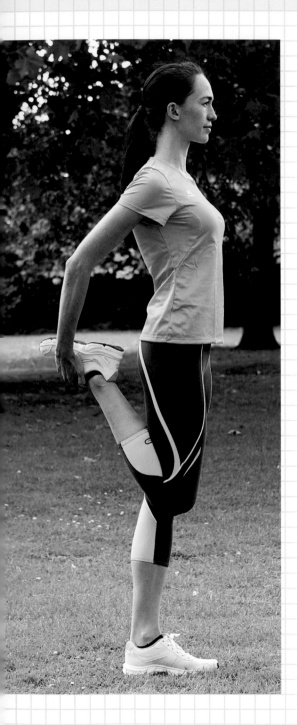

If you take just one thing from this chapter, let it be the all-important exercise that is the Stork. It's not only great for activating and strengthening your feet, ankles, and lower legs, it's excellent for your balance, something we tend to lose with age.

The best thing about the Stork is that it can be done anywhere and at any time—while you wait for a bus, while in line at the supermarket, or even at home in front of the television. There are no excuses for skipping your Storks. You must do them every day, without fail.

Tips

- For all variations, begin by standing barefoot on a clean, flat surface. Make sure it's a clear space with no furniture or walls within easy reach, so you're not tempted to grab onto them if you lose your balance.
- The goal is to hold your balance and avoid placing your foot back onto the floor. You can do this by holding your foot in your hand or, if you find that difficult, you can try step 2, or variation 2, opposite.

- If you lose your balance, hop around until you regain it. If you still find yourself wobbling, concentrate on your big toe and keep your eyes fixed on one object in the room. This will help you regain your balance.

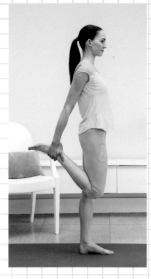

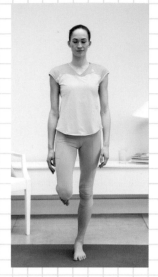

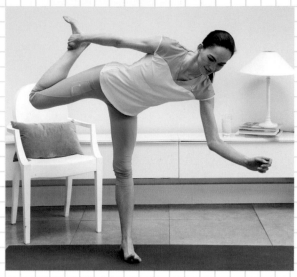

1 Lift one foot off the floor and hold it behind you. Try to hold for 15 seconds before switching to the other foot. Switch back and forth five times. You may find it easier to balance on one leg than the other. Make a mental note of which side of your body seems to function better.

2 Raise your foot behind you, without grabbing it with your hand.

Variation 1

If this exercise starts to get easy for you, challenge yourself by closing your eyes, or deliberately throwing yourself off balance by moving your body around in random directions. Feel your foot working to get the balance back.

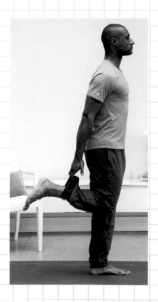

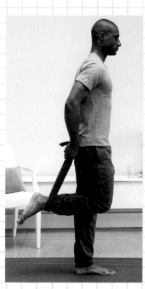

Variation 2

Hold on to the cuff of your trousers; or loop a yoga belt or cord around your ankle and hold it up behind you.

Work up to a full minute per leg until you're Storking for 10 minutes per day—that's 5 x (1:00 right foot/ 1:00 left foot).

How do you care for your feet?

If you'd like some insights into the male versus female psyche, ask the question, "How do you care for your feet?" Our female runners had a lot to say about how they felt about their trotters. Our male runners didn't seem to spare much thought for those things at the end of their ankles.

My feet are narrow and hard to fit into some kinds of shoes, but they do the job of hauling me around relatively uncomplainingly. MARY, SOUTH AFRICA

I clip my toenails when my wife starts complaining about them. PETER, USA

I limit myself to using a pumice stone every once in awhile. CLAUDIO, ITALY

I once got told I had feet like a Botticelli angel, which I took as a massive compliment...right up to the time I actually looked at the feet of a Botticelli angel. They're pudgy with tiny stubby toes. So yes, they really do look like mine! JOANNA, AUSTRALIA

I'm 5'9" and my poor size-seven feet have taken a beating over the years. As I've grown older, I've traded in my cute, uncomfortable heels for more comfortable, not so cute shoes. Doesn't do much for my "look," but has done wonders for my feet and even my knees. JEAN, UK

Never been a big fan of mine! But my ballet teachers used to love my high arches. And now I'm running I promise to be more thankful for their functionality. KELLY, IRELAND

My feet are the one body part about which I have never spoken negatively. They are not pretty, but I have always been rather grateful that they have been willing to carry me along—no matter how much I have weighed. TRACY, USA

Week 2 superstar profile: Jo Chapple

Age: 33
Location: New South Wales, Australia
Occupation: Teacher

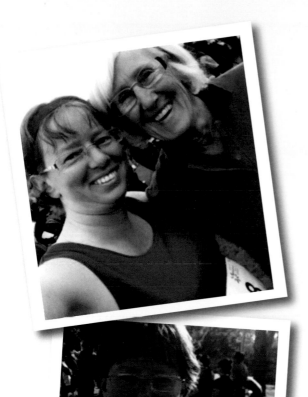

I didn't like sports as a kid. I saw exercise as a form of punishment and that view continued into my adult life. But I was tempted when I heard about Up & Running. I was tired of existing inside a blob instead of a body. The idea of being a runner was intriguing, even though it sounded impossible.

I was about 200lb when I started running and have recently reached my goal of being comfortably in my healthy weight range at 130lb. It was a slow but steady process and I think it helped that I didn't see weight loss as the sole purpose of my running, though of course I hoped that as I got healthier it would mean being lighter too. My new muscles amaze me. Having a strong body makes me feel stronger in other parts of my life as well.

Through running, I've proved to myself that I can make the choice to stick with something despite the ups and downs, and despite it often feeling not easy.

A huge lesson I had to learn was patience. This isn't something that I could swoop in and pick up in five minutes. I couldn't even spend long nights studying hard to get really good at it. I just had to keep on showing up for workouts and give my body time to adapt and learn.

Finishing my first 5k race was a highlight. Three years on, I've now run a half marathon and I'm training for another. My dreams have grown as my mind and body adapted to this new version of me. In all this time nothing has ever gone perfectly to plan when I've trained for a specific race or new distance, but I've learned that perfection is unnecessary and if I just keep showing up, then amazing things can happen.

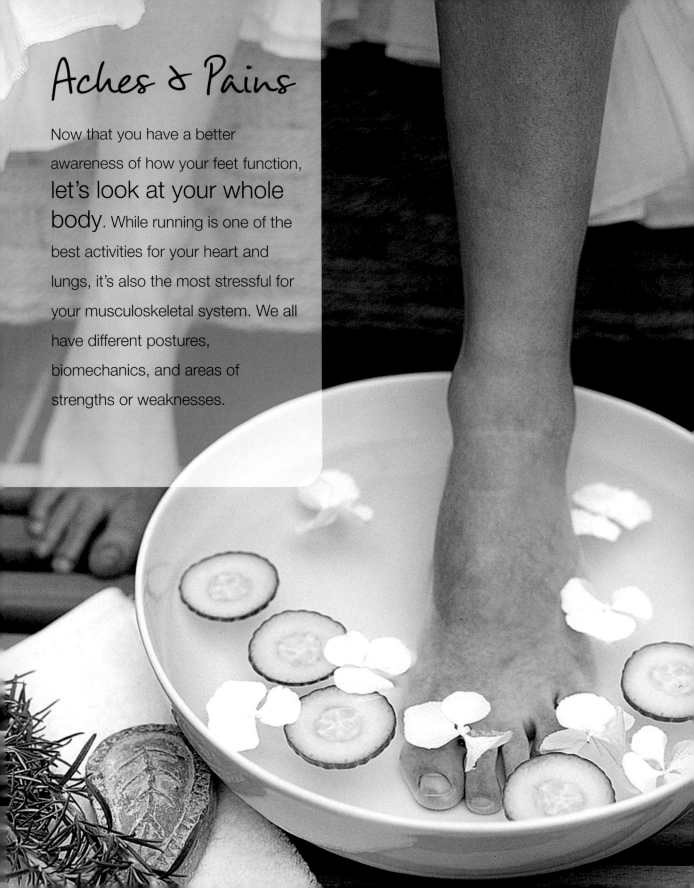

Aches & Pains

Now that you have a better awareness of how your feet function, **let's look at your whole body.** While running is one of the best activities for your heart and lungs, it's also the most stressful for your musculoskeletal system. We all have different postures, biomechanics, and areas of strengths or weaknesses.

We don't foresee any serious injuries during your 5k training, as your mileage is relatively low. If you've not exercised for a while, you may get some initial aches and pains but don't worry. Your body will adapt over time. The program is designed so that the distance and intensity gradually increase as you progress through the weeks, allowing your body to adapt slowly and your muscles to get stronger.

There are a few beginners' issues that are not major injuries, more small annoyances. You may encounter:

Shin Pain

Shin pain, or tibial stress, is the most common beginners' ailment. It's caused by unconditioned muscles being called into action. Your shins (or tibial muscles) are moved by your feet. When you start running, you're moving your feet in a new way, which may bring on some initial discomfort.

SOLUTION: Shin pain usually disappears once your muscles are warmed up. Stretch them out by rotating your ankles. Walk for a few minutes before you try running again. Repeat as many times as you need to. You can also ice your shins for 15 minutes a day and lightly massage them with arnica oil, an excellent anti-inflammatory. And above all, make sure you're doing your foot activation exercises every day. Get Storking!

Chafing

Chafing can occur where skin meets skin or where skin rubs against fabric. The most common points are between the thighs, under your armpits, on your nipples (both men and women), and beneath bra straps.

SOLUTION: Apply a thin layer of petroleum jelly or lubricant to the above-mentioned areas before your run. Wear compression shorts or running leggings to avoid thigh rub.

Muscle Fatigue/Good vs Bad Pain

Don't worry if your muscles are aching the day after a run. This is very common, caused by micro lesions forming on muscle fibers when these are stimulated or used in a different way. The aches normally disappear in a day or two, but if you've overexercised, it might take up to a week. This is why it's important to follow the training plan in sequence, to allow your muscles to get stronger and adapt to the gradually increased volume and intensity.

Muscle fatigue is a "useful" kind of soreness—it lets you know that your training is having an effect. But how can you tell if it's something more? "Useful" soreness is:

1. Bilateral (both the right and the left side should feel the same)
2. Constant (the same level of soreness, not increasing)
3. Absorbable (disappearing within a day or two)

Any pain outside of this description has to be examined more carefully.

SOLUTION: To relieve muscle fatigue, take a warm bath with Epsom salts. Many professional athletes in cold climates plunge their legs into ice-cold water. You could bathe your legs in a tub of ice cubes and cold water.

Damaged Toenails

Beneath the socks of many runners lurks the dreaded black toenail. This injury is more common if you run on irregular pavement or hills. All that up and down motion means your toes repeatedly hit against the upper toe box of your shoes. Toenails can also be damaged when your shoes don't fit properly (too much or too little room) or if they're not yet broken in.

SOLUTION: Keep your toenails clipped short. Make sure your shoes are the correct size. As we mentioned in the Warm-Up chapter, running shoes often need to be one size larger than your everyday shoes. When you have a new pair, break them in with a few walks before you take them on a running workout.

Blisters

Blisters form when skin overheats at a point of friction with your shoes or a point where there's too much pressure. You can get blisters with a new pair of shoes, by running too much too soon, or from wet socks rubbing against your skin during a rainy run.

The blister may fill up with fluid where the layers of skin separate. With deeper trauma it may even fill with blood, which is why you get a black blister. If you take care of blisters right away, you could be running again the very next day.

SOLUTION: Small blisters may disappear without issue. If it's a whopper, you may need to drain it with a sterile needle. Don't tear the skin; just make a small hole and drain the liquid. Air it out to dry the blistered skin. You can still run, but cover the blister with a regular plaster or a product that acts as a second skin while the blister heals.

Athlete's Foot

Athlete's foot is caused by a microscopic fungus that settles in between your toes. It's often picked up from gym locker-room floors, communal showers, and swimming pools. It begins with irritation on the soles of your feet or between your toes and can quickly develop into itching and unpleasant odor. It's aggravated by excessive sweating or shoes made with rubber (such as rubber sandals or clogs).

SOLUTION: Foot baths with antifungal salts along with a topical antifungal cream should quickly take care of the problem. Be sure to change your socks after every workout and air out your shoes by removing the inner soles and allowing them to dry.

Runner's Trots

It's very common to have intestinal problems while you run. Running can aid intestinal movement and help you to become more regular, but at other times it can contribute to stomach cramps, gas, nausea, and diarrhea. Unfortunately, it often happens halfway through a workout, in the middle of nowhere, with no restroom in sight.

SOLUTION: If you're having intestinal problems during your workouts, make sure you're taking in enough fluids throughout the day to avoid dehydration. Try to identify what foods trigger your digestive issues.

Common culprits are dairy products, yeast, and foods rich in sugar and/or fat. Caffeine can also speed up intestinal movement so you might want to try cutting down your intake.

You can also experiment with your workout times to make sure they don't coincide with your daily visit to the bathroom.

Cramps and Muscle Spasms

Cramps or continuous involuntary muscle spasms can last from a few seconds up to a full minute. They tend to occur if you're dehydrated or mineral deficient (potassium, calcium, magnesium, and/or phosphorus). Excessive heat or cold can also start them off. They're also common if you have tight muscles, so be sure to do your stretches.

SOLUTION: Cramps or muscle spasms don't generate any risk for the integrity of the muscle, although they may leave you feeling sore for a day or two. To prevent cramps occurring in the first place, keep flexible with regular yoga, Pilates, or stretching sessions. Eat plenty of fresh fruit and vegetables, which are good sources of vitamins and minerals; and drink plenty of water in small sips throughout the day, especially when the temperature rises.

Calluses

Calluses are areas of hard, thickened skin that develop when the skin is exposed to excessive pressure or friction. They're common on the soles of the feet, around the big and little toes, and on the heels. You may develop such thick calluses that they start to crack and break. Don't let it get that far.

SOLUTION: Prepare a basin with warm water and Epsom salts. Soak your feet for 10 minutes to soften the skin. Dab your feet dry, leaving them a little damp, then use a pumice stone to remove any excess skin. Before going to bed, apply a moisturizing cream. You could then put on a pair of socks and leave them on all night. They'll help your feet to absorb the cream and you'll have soft feet in the morning.

Week 2
Training Plan

- Free Form Walk with arm swings — 5:00
- Stretch — 3:00
- 6 x (walk 1:00/5 heel lifts) — 7:00
- 5 x (walk 1:00/slow run 0:30) — 7:30
- 1 km Free Form Run

Instructions

1 **Free Form Walk with arm swings**
Walk at a brisk pace for five minutes. Warm up your arms and shoulders by bending your elbows at a 90-degree angle and swinging them back and forth as you walk.

2 **Stretch**
Take three minutes to stop for a good stretch. Check out our stretch routine in the Warm-Up chapter.

Create time
You will never find the time to go running. Make the time. Plan your training sessions in advance and stick to your schedule.

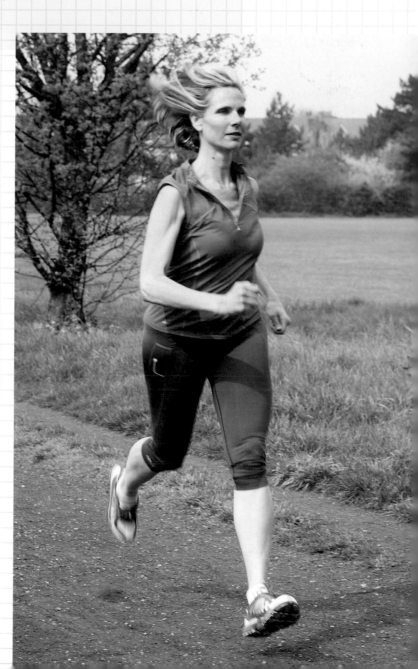

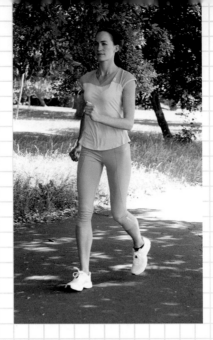

3 6 x (walk 1:00/5 heel lifts)

Walk for one minute then stop. Standing in place, lift your heels and rise up on the balls of your feet. Lower your heels and repeat four more times. Perform this walking/foot exercise circuit six times in total.

4 5 x (walk 1:00/ slow run 0:30)

Walk for one minute then run slowly for 30 seconds. Do this circuit five times in total.

5 1km Free Form Run

Remember that Free Form Running can be a combination of running and walking. Be sure to make a note of your 1km time.

When to train

Tuesday/Thursday/Saturday or Monday/Wednesday/Friday are ideal training days. You can do back to back days if you really need to, but avoid running three days in a row. Your body and muscles need recovery time.

Week 2 Wisdom

Run One—felt great next day. Run Two—a little bit tired next day. Run Three—EVERYTHING below the waist hurt, especially my buttocks! Here's hoping for the peachiest buns after eight weeks! PAULA, UK

Treadmill Modifications

- For the arm swings, choose a version that allows you to maintain your balance.
- Hop off the treadmill for stretching and the heel lifts.

Week 2 Exercise
Heel Lifts

Strong calf and foot muscles are a runner's best friends, and heel lifts are the perfect exercise to build them. Simply lifting your heels and going up on your toes gets four muscles firing:

- The gastrocnemius is the visible muscle when you look at your calves. It originates at the femur behind the knee and attaches to the heel with the Achilles tendon.
- The soleus is hidden beneath the gastrocnemius on the lower part of the leg.
- The plantaris runs obliquely and lies between the soleus and the medial head of the gastrocnemius.
- The plantar fascia is not actually a muscle but a thick cord of connective tissue that runs from your heel to your metatarsal bones, supporting the arch of your foot.

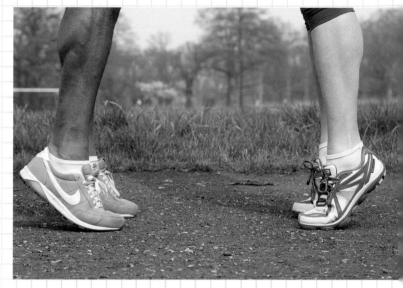

To perform heel lifts, put your hands on your hips or stretch them straight out in front of you for balance. Rise up on the balls of your feet, then lower your heels back down. You don't need to stay up on your toes for more than a split second.

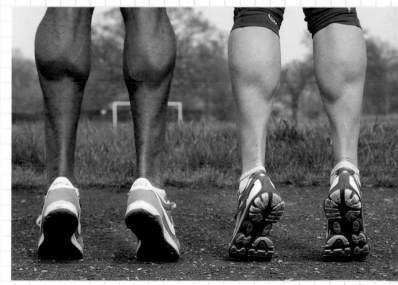

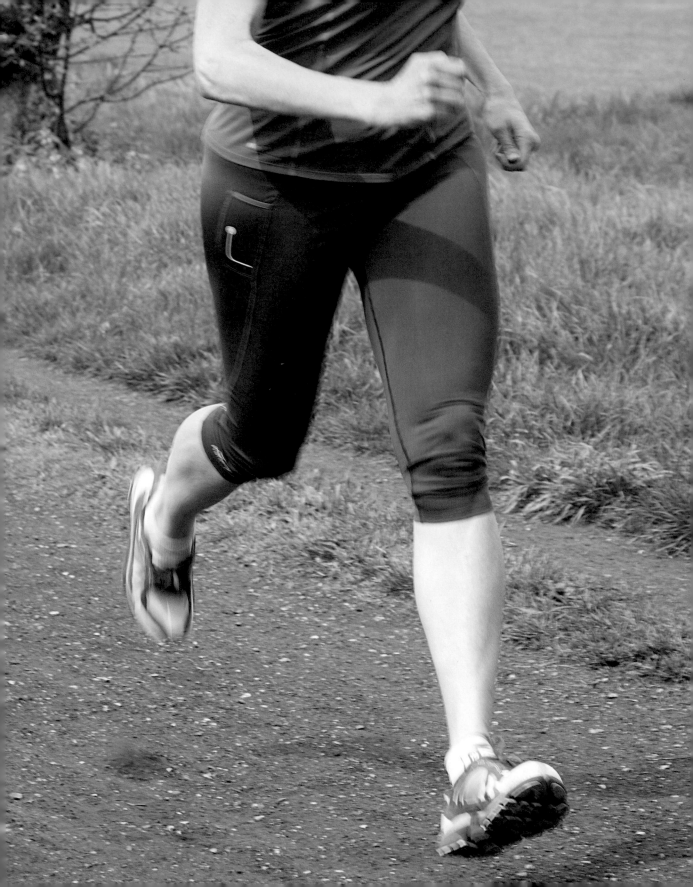

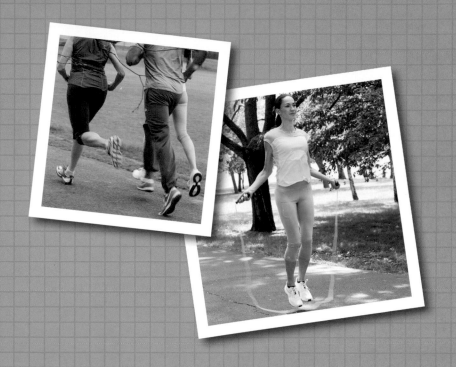

Staying the Course

Staying Motivated

Most people don't make just one attempt to become runners. Many try a training plan three, four, even ten times, starting **strong** but never quite hitting their goal of racing that 5k. Like New Year's resolutions, **reality** sets in once the champagne glass is empty and the fireworks have faded. Achieving your goals is not as easy as lying on the couch and dreaming about them.

When people struggle to complete the 5k program, they usually put it down to a lack of effort. But most often there's more to it. It's because we get in our own way.

Do any of these sound familiar?

If you're **overexcited**, you start out with bubbly, contagious enthusiasm. But as the weeks go by and the initial adrenaline rush of a new project dissolves, your eagerness for your workouts wanes, too.

SOLUTION: Refocus right before you go out the door for each and every workout. Close your eyes and imagine the buzz you'll feel when you start running. Now, go!

If you're **overambitious**, you're impatient to get things started. You've glanced over the training plan and think that you can skip weeks one through four and condense this into a one-month program. How about a marathon plan instead?

SOLUTION: Your mind and spirit may be ready for endurance sports but your body needs time to adapt physiologically to your new running routine. Give it the time it deserves. If you want to speed up the process, be extra vigilant with post-run recovery—pay attention to your nutrition and sleep quality. Once you've laid down a solid foundation, you can risk running harder, faster, and longer.

Overprocessers need to think about running *every single step of the way*. You leave little room for spontaneity and before you even put on your running shoes, you're doubting your choice of model. Maybe you should go back to the store?

SOLUTION: Don't think, run! Remind yourself that this is an excellent opportunity to practice going with the flow in 45-minute increments. Follow the instructions each week, as written. Deep breaths!

If you're a **perfectionist**, you frequently start and stop your training, then start all over again from Week 1. Everything has to be *just so*. Your workout app didn't pick up a satellite signal and didn't correctly measure the distances you covered. Now you're not sure if you really ran for a full kilometer. This devastating lack of data leaves you convinced that your only option is to start the whole program again. And again, because something else is bound to go awry and be less than absolute *perfection*.

SOLUTION: Besides the obvious sweat and dirt involved, running is a messy activity. The numbers don't always add up correctly and technical hitches are inevitable. But if you've stepped out the door, moved around and clocked some time, this is definitely considered a workout. Remember that saying, "perfect is the enemy of done."

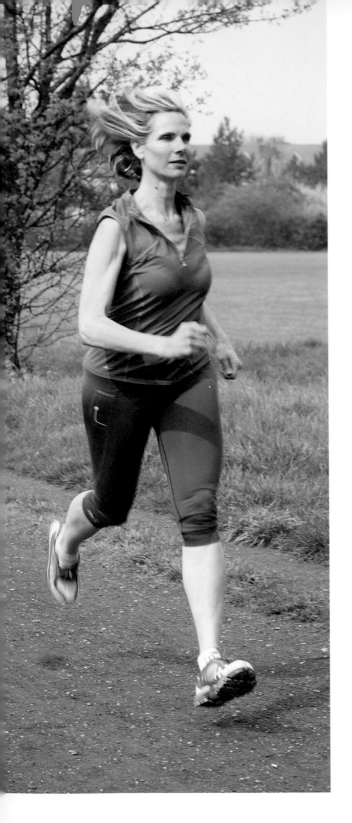

Why the First 20 Minutes of Your Run are Always the Hardest

You may have had a vision of how your runs would feel. You'd trot outside and feel the breeze on your face. Your legs would glide effortlessly along the road. You'd be at one with nature and your body would buzz with that famous runner's high.

But in reality? Your lungs are burning, your legs feel like lead, and you're gasping for breath.

If that sounds like your experience, you're probably in the first 20 minutes of your workout.

The body takes time to warm up. It's a process that begins even as you're lacing up your shoes. First the heart starts to pump faster. As you begin your arm circles, the blood begins to flow faster and circulates to the extremities of your body. Your body temperature begins to rise, which warms up your muscles and makes them more pliable.

Those first running steps may feel awkward. This is because your body needs to adapt to the movement. No matter what your fitness level or running experience, you will go through this process. It's an individual thing; for some it may even take half an hour or more.

But on average, the first 20 minutes of a run **are pretty hard** for absolute beginners and élite runners alike. So please understand that it's perfectly normal to feel awful in those first 20 minutes and that you're in good company. The runner's high will make its appearance once your body is properly warmed up.

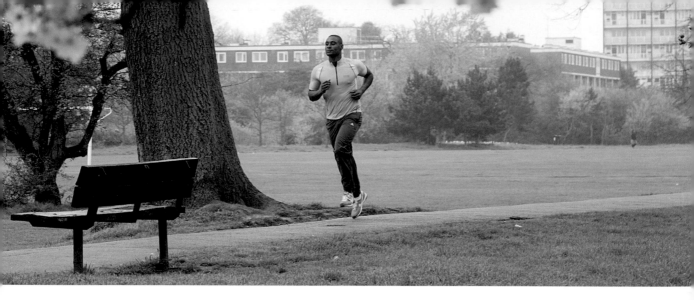

Nobody Pays Attention to You When You Run

This is the wholehearted and honest advice we've always given our 5k course runners as they nervously lace up their shoes for their first training session. And now we're going to tell you the same thing.

We know it's easier said than done. It's been the number one Week 1 worry expressed by our 5k runners over the years. The logical part of our brains is easily overpowered by the part that's paranoid about the size of our bums, our sweaty red faces, and/or our glacial pace. There may be traumatic memories of being laughed at in PE class. You may fear that someone from work will see you.

But we promise you that for the most part, people are lost in their own thoughts and will not even notice you. And if they do, most will think, "Dang, I really need to do some exercise."

We humans are a self-absorbed species. That skinny runner with the swishy ponytail is probably not frowning at your running technique; she's more likely worried about a big meeting or child-transport logistics. That guy with the amazing calf muscles who's going really fast is not scoffing at your slowness; he's busy visualizing his next marathon PB. Those teenaged boys who seem to be smirking your way at the park? Just

think about their pimples and squeaky voices and feel sorry for them.

Let's face it, genuinely bitchy folks do exist. A relative of Shauna's, who shall remain nameless, once said, "Yes she may be a successful doctor, but she's got very thick ankles." There is nothing you can do about these kinds of people. Doing something new requires courage. It requires busting out of our comfort zone and allowing ourselves to be seen. We are only asking you to be brave for 40 minutes, three times a week. You can do this.

Put on some banging tunes while you get dressed. Mentally run through your motivations to remember why you're doing this instead of hiding on the couch.

If you're feeling particularly fragile, deploy Shauna's **vampire method**—that is, do your workout as early in the day as is safe to do so. At those hours, you'll mostly see hardcore runners and they tend to give a friendly nod to anyone crazy enough to be awake…or they'll ignore you completely.

Be brave and get out there, regardless of who's watching. In the end, this is your life and your health. We know it can be hard at times, but hard is where the magic happens.

How do You Feel About Running in Public?

Overcoming any reservations about running in public is a big step toward enjoying the training plan. The more you run outside, the easier it becomes!

There's a flurry of thoughts running through my head: I hope my stomach doesn't show too much, maybe I should have put on the XL shirt, look at that guy running faster than me, if I start skipping now are they going to think I'm crazy?

ALESSIO, ITALY

In the beginning, I wore headphones, wouldn't make eye contact, and took "private" routes for the potentially more embarrassing drills. It's hard being confident when you're red-faced, out of breath, and feeling slow. It got easier as my running improved. Or more accurately: as I saw myself more as a "real" runner. I also realized most people aren't looking at all.

TESSA, NETHERLANDS

I'm an exhibitionist and getting attention from others gives me energy and enthusiasm. In exchange, I try to offer others a vision of a fun, happy runner.

ENOLLIS, GREECE

When I first started running, I dressed in a sober manner so I wouldn't be noticed. No special running gear, no flashy sunglasses. But then I got over it and now I wear whatever I want without worrying about what others may think of me. I'm proud to be a runner. BEPI, ITALY

My general line of thinking starts with "Oh God, what will people think?" and ends up at "Who cares! If they don't like my butt, that's their problem. Plenty of world around here, look at something else." I've only ever encountered one person I knew. We stopped and chatted for a minute then went on our merry ways. The funny thing is, if you see someone while you're out exercising, they may well be exercising too! It puts you on an even playing field, even if you are sweaty and red-faced. BELLA, AUSTRALIA

Week 3 superstar profile:
Matteo Panini

Age: 43
Location: Modena, Italy
Occupation: Organic farmer

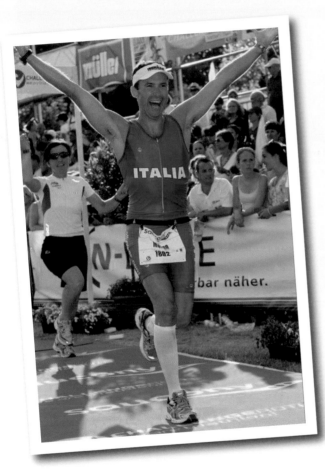

Before running, I raced cars. Any other sport was solely practiced in order to maintain my fitness and to help me drive better and faster.

The running spark was lit with the birth of my first daughter, Valentina. We have a summer house in the Dolomite Mountains and in the afternoons I started going out for a ride on my mountain bike. After a month, besides losing a few unwanted pounds, I felt great. When I returned home, I began running to maintain my fitness. I love numbers, so the stopwatch played a big part in capturing my interest. Before I knew it, I was passionate about running.

Julia's training methods opened up a whole new world. They weren't the usual training plans; they had a constant muscle-strengthening path, which led me from 5k all the way up to my first marathon.

Everyone knows that I'm unavailable at lunchtime from 1pm to 3pm. It's a choice I made and I have to say that these running breaks have given me a better quality of life.

I struggle to get myself ready for a run, but I'm lucky to be in the countryside with lots of beautiful trails. I love running out of the city where there's less traffic. After a run, I have a feeling of widespread wellbeing throughout my body.

The most beautiful race I've ever run was the 100k of Sahara in Tunisia in 2004. I have wonderful memories of beautiful Tunisian landscapes and an excellent personal performance (I finished in 28th place out of 150 competitors).

My advice to new runners? Start out calmly, because the road is long. Remember that there will always be someone faster than you, but there will also be those who are slower than you, too.

Week 3
Training Plan

- Free Form Walk with arm swings — 5:00
- Stretch — 3:00
- 5 x (skip 0:15/walk 0:45) — 5:00
- 5 x (slow run 0:30/slow walk 0:15/fast walk 0:15) — 5:00
- 2 x 1km Free Form Run (5:00 recovery in between)

Instructions

1 Free Form Walk with arm swings
Begin with a brisk five-minute walk with full-circle arm swings. Bring your arms up over your head and then back again in the opposite direction.

2 Stretch
Take three minutes to stop for a good stretch.

3 5 x (skip 0:15/walk 0:45)
Skip for 15 seconds and then walk for 45 seconds for a total of five circuits. Make sure you pump your arms to help your balance and rhythm.

Keep a training diary
Seeing your times improve week after week will keep you motivated.

Week 3 Wisdom
Let me tell you, this town is crazy busy at 5am. I thought I'd be skipping my little heart out with no onlookers. No chance. The route I chose was also chosen by a random man walking to work. I was more than happy to provide him with entertainment in the form of arm swings and skipping. It's my little way of bringing smiles to the faces of the "walking to work at 5am" set. AMY, USA

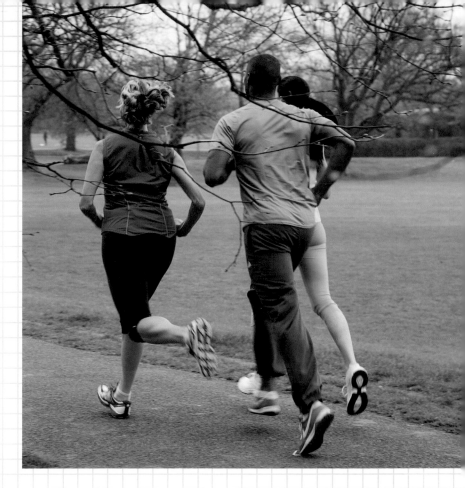

4   5 x (slow run 0:30/ slow walk 0:15/fast walk 0:15)

As you repeat this slow run > slow walk > fast walk circuit, feel the flow from one mode to the next. Start to learn that you have more than one running gear.

Track your mileage
This is another great way to gauge your progress.

5   2 x 1km Free Form Run (5:00 recovery in between)

We've doubled your running time this week. You have a five-minute recovery time between the two 1km runs. Use that time to stretch, catch your breath, or walk around a little. Take it easy on the first 1km so you have energy left for the second.

Treadmill Modifications

- For the arm swings, choose a version that allows you to maintain your balance.
- Hop off the treadmill for stretching.
- Do the entire skip/walk sequence off the treadmill. The skipping can be done in a nearby corridor, then walk around for 45 seconds before repeating the sequence.

Week 3 Exercise
Skipping

Skipping is a basic drill that even élite athletes practice on a regular basis. Keep this in mind if you feel shy about skipping in a public setting.

The forward skipping movement gently encourages you to activate your feet and ankles, and lift your knees. Skipping is one of the best exercises for runners who tend to "shuffle" since it forces you to use your feet in order to move forward. While performing your skipping drills remember:

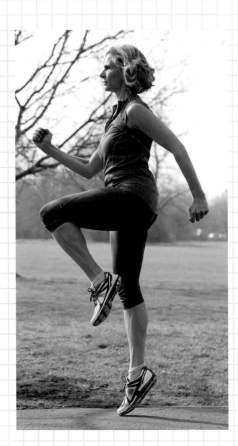

Start with your elbows bent at a 90-degree angle with your hands closed but not clenched.

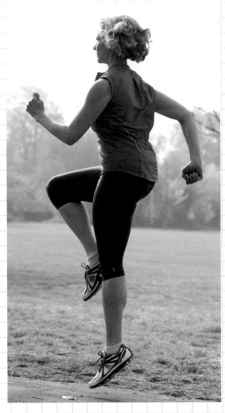

Use your arms for balance and "lift–off." Synchronize your arms with your skips: left leg lifts together with your right arm; right leg with your left arm.

Tips
- Push yourself forward, not up.
- Concentrate on your feet. Feel them pushing off the ground in a forward motion.

Week 3 Exercise
Learning to Judge Speed

Your Week 3 training contains a circuit of slow run > slow walk > fast walk, which will help you learn about your different speeds.

The ability to gauge speed is one of the most difficult skills for any runner to learn, no matter how much experience they have. When novice athletes start running, they usually think, "fast." But running has many different speeds, from slow to moderate to fast, steady state to progressive, with many variations on all of them.

People have their own speed and it varies enormously from one person to the next. Your slow run is going to be different from Kara Goucher's slow run. It doesn't matter how fast your pace is because it will change over time. The important thing is to learn to feel your speed, and how to shift it up and down as if you had gears.

The easiest way to begin this process is by first paying attention to the difference between your slow walk and fast walk.

Slow walking is slow walking; there is no better definition. But to go from slow walking to fast walking there are two movements you need to concentrate on:

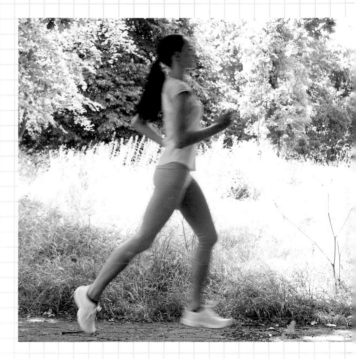

1. **Shortening your stride (the length of your steps)**
2. **Increasing your leg turnover or cadence (how fast your legs are moving)**

Most people make the mistake of taking bigger steps when they want to walk or run faster. This makes their stride longer and slows down their cadence. Not only does this put more stress on hips and knees, it's an inefficient way to walk and run because it quickly fatigues the muscles.

Instead, we recommend that you begin by concentrating on increasing your leg turnover. This will automatically shorten your stride. Use your arms, elbows at a 90-degree angle, to give yourself rhythm and balance.

To transition from a fast walk to a slow run, simply use your feet to push off the ground. Then, to go from a slow run to a faster run, once again concentrate on increasing your leg turnover and keeping your stride short. It's that simple.

This whole exercise will not feel natural at first. But in time you'll get a feel for it and see that it allows you to move faster, more easily, and with less chance of injury.

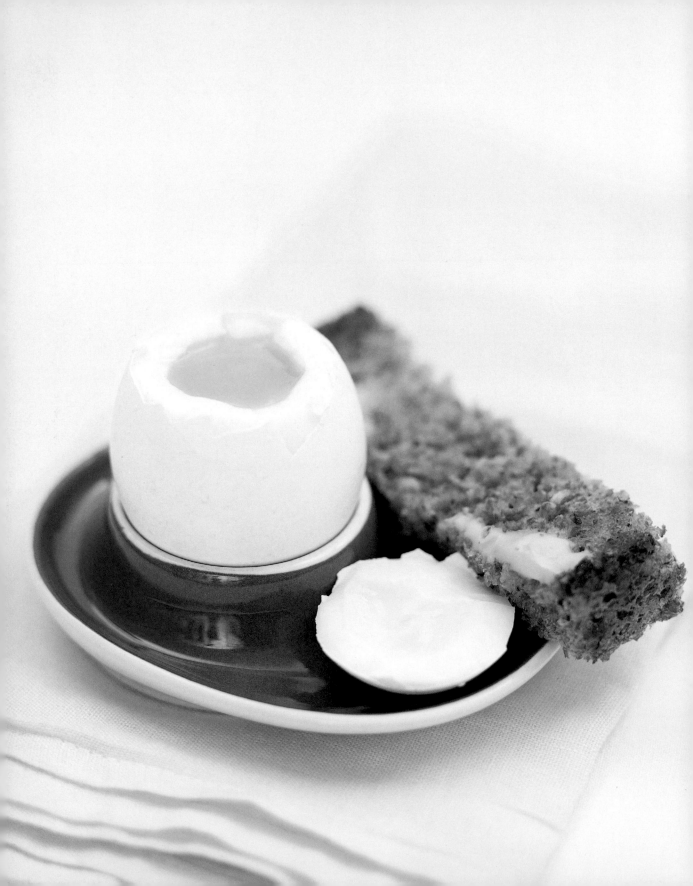

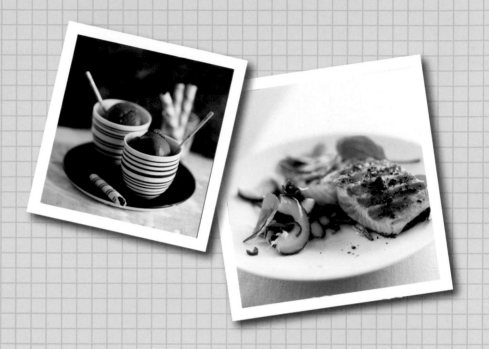

Food as Fuel

Fuelling Your Run

If you want to see how crazy the western world has become about food, just flip on the television.

On the one hand, there's a plethora of competitive cooking shows and glamorous celebrity chefs whipping up rich, fancy, and delicately "plated" food. In contrast are the diet programs, berating people for their food choices and shaming them back into shape.

Somewhere along the way we've lost sight of what food is meant to be: nourishment, pleasure, and, above all, fuel for our bodies.

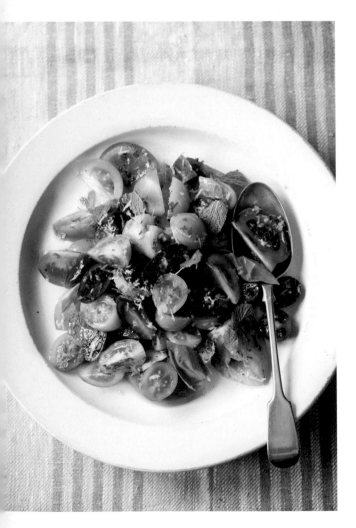

The quality and quantity of the food you consume has an impact on your health and well-being, not to mention your running. We don't advocate any one specific way of eating. We believe that each individual has to find what nutrition plan works best for his or her body.

This depends on a multitude of factors. Age, gender, and hormones will influence how your food is processed and metabolized. Some of you may choose the Paleo path, whereas others have their roots deeply planted in the vegan world (no pun intended). There is no right or wrong way. But if you have fitness or running goals, you need to start examining your eating habits and figure out what works best for you. Which foods supply you with more energy to run but also keep the scale on an even keel?

Tomatoes are an excellent source of the antioxidant lycopene, which is important for both skin and bone.

Clean Up Your Diet

Start by looking at food quality. It may not have a huge effect on your training and your first 5k race, but now is a great time to begin working on your nutrition, both for your long-term health and future running ambitions. Forget "diets" and extreme changes; start by making small tweaks.

Eliminate Excess Sugar

Sugar is completely devoid of nutrition. It contains no vitamins or minerals, only empty calories. It might give you a quick hit of energy, but on the downside it can play havoc with your blood-sugar levels. That's not good for anyone, let alone an athlete.

Unfortunately, sugar lurks in many products, some of which you may not suspect, such as bread, yogurt, processed meat, and cereals. Your body becomes accustomed to that sugar hit and puts you on a wild glycemic rollercoaster ride all day.

It's easy to eliminate excess sugar from your diet—just learn to read food labels. Sugar can come in many forms, such as corn syrup, rice syrup, dextrose, maltose, fructose, lactose, or raw sugar. Once you've become a label-reading expert, start to wean yourself off sugar in your tea and coffee or any other daily consumption.

This doesn't mean you shouldn't eat sugar every once in a while as a treat. Life is short and chocolate truffle ice cream is almost orgasmic. When your daily diet is low in sugar, that dessert treat will be so much more delicious and special.

Eat your Grains Whole

Buy whole grain bread, pasta, and rice. The white versions have been stripped and bleached in the manufacturing process. Whole grains not only contain more protein and fiber, they taste better, too. This doesn't mean you need to skip the pizza on your vacation. Go ahead. But get back on the whole-grain train as soon as you get home.

Start your Main Meals with Raw Vegetables

Fresh vegetables are filling and full of vitamins and minerals. They'll keep your intestinal tract healthy and give you clear, healthy skin. Plus, they're good to eat. Prepare and chop salad items in advance and put them into a giant bowl. Our favorites include three or four types of lettuce, arugula, carrots, fennel, cucumbers, and tomatoes. Don't add the dressing yet. When mealtime comes around you have a beautiful salad ready to serve.

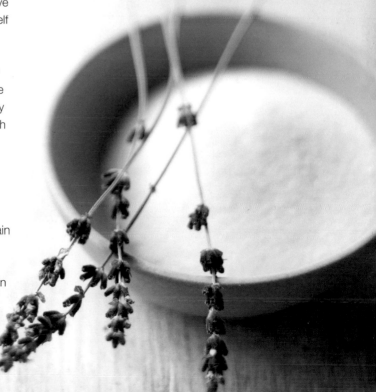

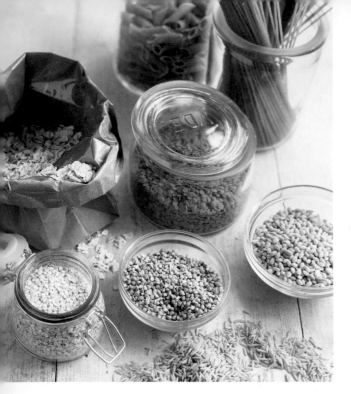

One last recommendation: eat your fruit and vegetables instead of drinking them. Concentrated juices are loaded with sugar, albeit natural ones. Your body will have an insulin response to a glass of orange juice as if it were a sugar-laden soda. If you're thirsty, drink a glass of water instead.

Balance Protein and Carbohydrates

The biggest myth for runners is that you need to eat more carbohydrates. That's why many marathon runners gain weight despite their grueling training schedules. Look for ways to include protein in your daily menu, such as an egg at breakfast and grilled fish or poultry at lunch or dinner. Beans and legumes have endless culinary possibilities. Use nuts and seeds sparingly. They're a delicious source of protein and healthy fats, but most of us don't know when to put them away.

ABOVE: Although you don't need to increase your intake of carbohydrates, slow-release carbs, such as whole grains, are absorbed slowly and keep your blood sugar at a steady level, which keeps hunger pangs away and stops you snacking between meals.

Don't feel like you have to change everything today, or even by next week. Pick one item from the list and stick to that for a while and see how your habits evolve. If you feel you need more guidance, make an appointment with a dietitian or qualified nutritionist.

Time your Meals along with your Workouts

Understanding the workings of your digestive system will benefit your running. Our bodies function uniquely, but we can roughly divide runners into two groups: those who can run on an empty stomach and those who need some fuel to get going.

If you're doing your workouts first thing in the morning but can't exercise on an empty stomach, try eating an easily digested food, such as a banana, and drinking a glass of water. This should get you through the run without giving you side stitches or intestinal problems. Looking forward to a complete breakfast after your workout might even help you get through it.

You can use the same fueling strategy if you're running during your lunch hour or later in the afternoon. Avoid running on a full stomach; so make sure you allow two to three hours to digest your previous meal. Again, experiment to see what works best for you.

Food FAQs

Q. Why does running make me so hungry?
A. Changing your routine can slightly rev up your appetite. It doesn't necessarily mean you need more calories. It's easy to overestimate "the burn" of your workouts, but if you're persistently hungrier, increase your fruit and vegetable intake and be sure to eat quality, nutrient-dense whole foods rather than processed foods that lack the satiety factor.

Q. What should I eat after a run?
A. First have a glass of water to make sure you're not mistaking hunger for thirst. If you're still hungry, have a piece of fruit. At your current training volume you mostly likely won't need to eat any more food than before you started the program.

Week 4 superstar profile:
Marci Gaither

Age: 41
Location: Pittsburgh, USA
Occupation: Psychologist

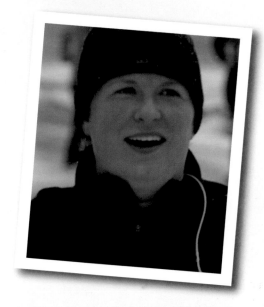

I always liked the idea of running. I wished I could be a runner, but didn't think I was cut out for it. I stumbled across Up & Running and in a moment of optimism I thought, "Why not?" and signed up.

I didn't think I could do it. I was afraid it would be just too hard for me. I don't look like the stereotypical runner, so was also a little self-conscious when starting my public workouts. I was amazed at the support I received. Complete strangers in the park stopped me to offer encouragement.

I was still not able to run a full 5k at the end of the eight weeks. Remember, I was SLOW and could only run about 30 seconds at a time when I started. But Julia said we had to try to complete a 5k for a base time, and by God, you learn to do what Julia tells you.

My first 5k race was not fun. I won't lie. I did it by myself because I felt I couldn't ask anyone to do it with me. No one else would be that slow. I also didn't learn about the route ahead of time and didn't realize it was a hilly one. I came in dead last. The guy was breaking down the finish chute when I came in. But I did it, and then had my base 5k time to work from.

I set my sights on the "Run The Whole 5k goal," and started by redoing the 5k training plan. Then Julia worked with me to suggest some modifications. And after many months of hard work, one day it came true. I ran the whole five kilometers.

As someone who practices cognitive behavioral therapy, I have learned how running is a perfect example of how important our thinking is to everything we do. And you have a lot of time to think when you run. Early on I declared my running time as a "no negativity zone." I try hard to keep my thoughts on encouraging, positive messages. I have learned that I am capable of more than I thought.

I frequently don't want to go. I'm much better now at catching myself early on when my thinking slides in the slacker direction. I tell myself that it is non-negotiable. I tell myself I will feel better afterward (this is always true). Sometimes, I tell myself, "Suck it up, cupcake!" I might pop onto the Up & Running Forum to see what others are up to and get motivated that way, too. And most of the time I'm meeting up with a running buddy, so we keep each other accountable.

I don't feel like a gazelle when I run, I'll tell you that. I'm usually reminding myself of various motivational phrases. I have a whole Pinterest board full of them. Sometimes I'm happy not to have to think about much of anything. I don't have to make any decisions. I just have to run. I listen to music when I run, too.

Even a crappy run feels good, because you're proud that you did it. The whole "a good mood is only a run away" thing is true.

I'm still running, farther than ever before. I rocked the Up & Running 10k Course. I can now run for eight miles at a time. Me! I have dropped through the rabbit hole. Anything is possible now.

Running and Weight Loss

You may have started running with the hope of shedding some pounds. You've heard that running burns more calories than any other activity. Your svelte runner friends brag about how they can eat anything they want. You want to believe!

The truth is that while running can aid weight loss, it's not a miracle cure. If fat loss is your goal, the single most important factor in determining your success will be your food intake.

If your scales are not showing a loss—or are even going up—there could be a number of different reasons:

Your Diet
Are you eating too much?
You may be overestimating the amount of food your body needs. We don't recommend calorie counting as a long-term solution, but tracking your food intake for just seven days can usually provide insights into why the scale is not shifting. Try a free smartphone app, such as Lose It! or MyFitnessPal. Also, keep an eye out for:

- Too many "treats" throughout the day
- A lack of fresh vegetables and fruit on your plate
- Any imbalance in your daily intake of macronutrients (carbohydrates, protein, and fat)

Are you eating too little?
Many people drastically reduce their food intake when trying to lose a few unwanted pounds, then wonder why they feel listless, tired, and unable to complete even the simplest workout. You may feel fine on a restricted regime for a few days, but it will catch up with you and inevitably propel you toward the nearest bakery. This has nothing to do with "willpower"—it's simply your body craving energy in the form of calories. Reducing your food intake too drastically will set you up on a roller-coaster ride with your weight, slow down your metabolism, and ultimately result in the opposite of your desired effect.

Your Incidental Movement Between Workouts
It's essential to look not only at your planned exercise but also at your incidental movement. We've met a lot of runners who were couch potatoes outside of their three weekly runs. Try wearing a pedometer for a few days and see how much you move. It's scary to see how few steps many of us take. Three 45-minute workouts will not make up for hours of sitting. If you want to get the scale moving, include as much everyday activity as you can.

DOMS and Fluid Retention
If you're feeling slightly sore, stiff, and achy the day after your workout, that's Delayed Onset of Muscle Soreness (DOMS). DOMS indicate a micro-tear in the muscle structure and a rupturing of muscle cells. Don't be alarmed—this is something you want to happen and your training is designed to have this effect. Your body will start repairing the damage and the muscle will be stronger after 24 to 48 hours.

But in order to repair the muscle, the body elicits an inflammatory response, which can cause fluid retention. The bad news: you may see the scale go up for a day or two. The good news: inflammation protects you from future muscle damage (also known as the Repeated Bout Effect), so over time you'll get less DOMS and be able to run longer, stronger, and with possibly less fluid retention.

Water Retention

Are your rings feeling tighter in the morning or your feet and ankles slightly swollen? Indulged in a Chinese takeaway or had salty popcorn at the movies? Ladies, is your period due soon? That extra pound on the scale could be water retention. Running can bring temporary relief from fluid retention by helping you sweat out some of the excess water.

You can also take care of this with food. Raw fennel is a great natural diuretic—grate it into salads or eat with your crudités. Unsweetened cranberry juice is a delicious choice for women who tend to retain water right around the time of their period. Try to use less salt for a day or two and see if that helps you "lose" the extra pound.

What You Actually Weigh

The scale is a good tool to monitor weight trends, but when you stare at that number in the morning light, remember what that number actually represents. Aside from fat, your body weight is also composed of muscles, bones, blood, and other bodily fluids. If any of these factors increase or decrease, so will the number on the scale.

A more useful number is your body fat percentage. You can have this professionally measured or purchase body fat scales. The readings are not always precise, but if you measure yourself consistently at the same time of day, you can track trends and gauge your progress.

If you belong to the "Scale Addicts Anonymous" Club, make sure you don't weigh yourself more than once a day, otherwise you're no longer monitoring fat loss but rather water-retention patterns. Plus, it's not good for your psyche!

If the scale isn't moving but you feel like you've lost inches, put on a snug pair of jeans or trousers. Use them as a measuring stick and note over time if they're easier or more difficult to zip up. Or, if you'd like more data, use a tape measure and regularly measure your waist, hips, and thighs.

Are your legs looking slimmer? Did you feel sexy before you got on the scale? If so, that extra pound is most likely a pound of muscle. That's great news because an extra pound of muscle will help you run better and increase your metabolism (that's why men burn more calories than women). Muscle is also denser than body fat, which is why your jeans are fitting better.

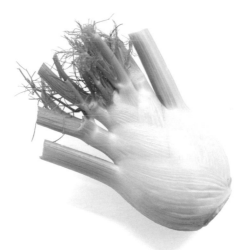

RIGHT: Raw fennel is an excellent natural diuretic and is easily added to salads. You could also enjoy it as a crudité.

Week 2
Training Plan

- Free Form Walk with arm swings — 5:00
- Stretch — 3:00
- 5 x (skip 0:15/walk 0:45/fast walk 0:30) — 7:30
- Rest — 2:00
- 6 x (0:30 run/1:00 walk) — 9:00
- 1.5km Free Form Run

Instructions

1 Free Form Walk with arm swings
Walk at a brisk pace for five minutes. Warm up your arms and shoulders by bending your elbows at a 90-degree angle and swinging them back and forth as you walk.

2 Stretch
Take three minutes to stop for a good stretch.

3 5 x (skip 0:15/walk 0:45/fast walk 0:30)
Start this circuit with 15 seconds of skipping then transition into a slow walk for 45 seconds. Now move into a fast walk for another 30 seconds. Feel the difference between a fast and a slow walk.

Don't watch the clock
You can time your intervals but don't look at the stopwatch while you're running. Just concentrate on covering the distance.

Week 4 Wisdom
Hours after my workout, I was walking across a parking lot when a thought popped into my head: *Wow, my legs feel really strong! Oh right, must be all that running. Brilliant!* This was a great realization, as one of my motivations from Warm-Up Week was to feel strong...jackpot! RORY, USA

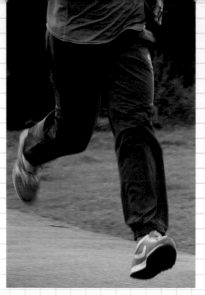
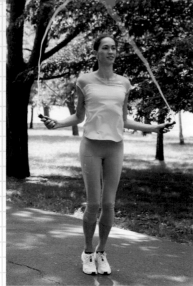

4 Rest
Take a two-minute break—
this can be stretching or slow
walking. If you feel ready to
continue, skip this break and
start the next exercise.

5 6 x (0:30 run/
1:00 walk)
Alternate running for 30
seconds with walking for one
minute for a total of six cycles.
Remember to run SLOWLY,
not fast.

6 1.5km Free Form Run
Run, walk, or do a mix of both
in whatever proportions you
want—whatever feels right at
that moment. Don't be afraid
to push yourself a little.

Look straight ahead
Avoid looking down at the
ground. Notice your thoughts.
If you notice any negative
ones popping into your head,
consciously turn your mind
to something positive.
Changing your thoughts can
help change your body
language and get you through
the workout.

Treadmill Modifications
- For the arm swings, choose a
  version that allows you to
  maintain your balance.
- Hop off the treadmill
  for stretching.
- Do the skip/walk/fast walk
  sequence off the treadmill.
  The skipping can be done in a
  corridor near the treadmill,
  then walk around for the
  walking segments.

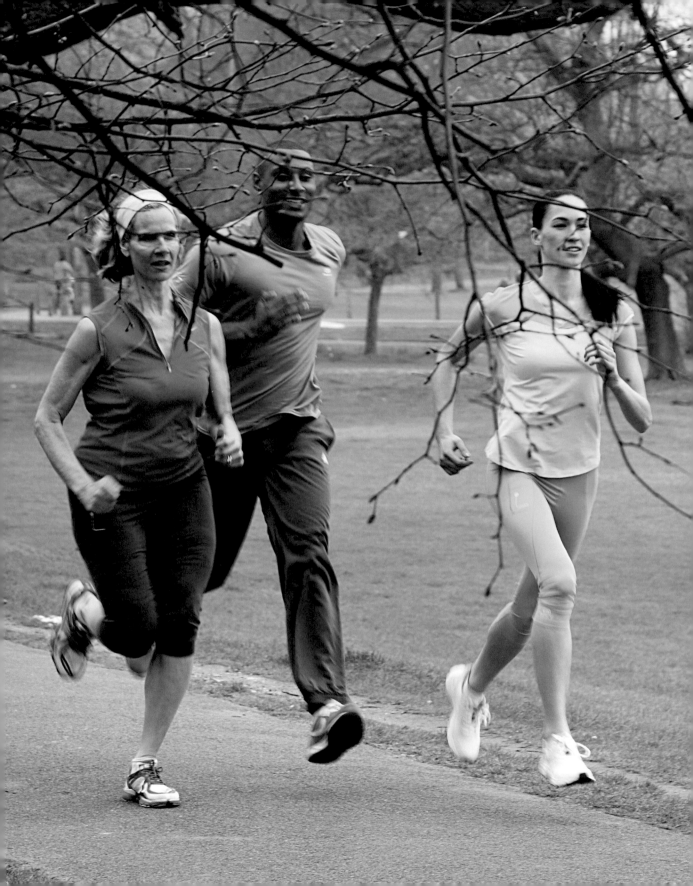

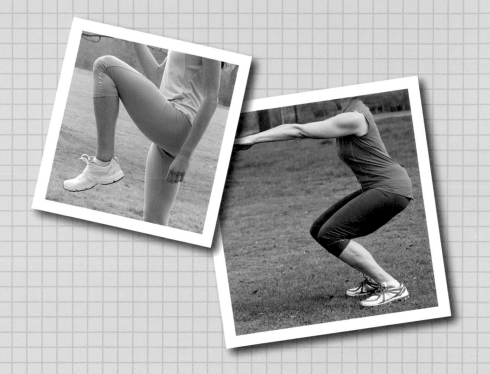

Halftime Check-In

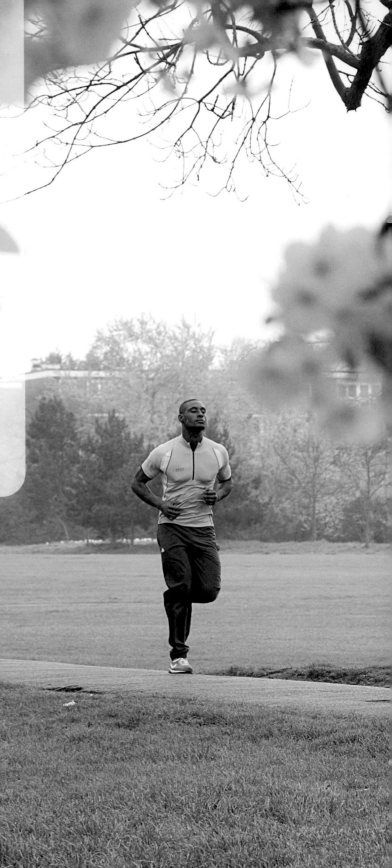

The Halfway Point

Before Shauna began running, she was one of those people who always started projects but never finished them. **Beginnings** are so much **fun**—especially when they involve new stationery. Surely a fresh, shiny training **diary** means amazing things are going to happen?!

Of course, after the thrill of starting something new comes a load of hard work, followed swiftly by self-doubt, critical thoughts, and a resigned feeling of "maybe this isn't meant to be?"

Shauna's running adventure started just like that. She did each run with her husband, who bravely endured her thrice-weekly whining. "This is really hard. Why is Julia making me skip? My shins hurt. Who put that hill there? This was a stupid idea," until the heavy breathing took over and she no longer had enough energy to complain.

Somehow she kept going. A lot of it was fear of disappointing Julia—there is something about the woman that shone a light on Shauna's flimsy excuses and made her dig deep. But mostly she wanted to finish those eight weeks for herself. She wanted to be one of those people who say they're going to do something then do it.

And she did. When she crossed the finish line at her 5k race, she bawled like a baby. After years of writing herself off for being too big, too unfit, too unworthy, she'd taken her body to a place she never thought it could go. She'd stuck it out for 24 workouts and finally finished something.

Keep the Momentum Going

We want you to know that feeling, too. You're now halfway through your 5k training—congratulations on making it this far. As we head into the final 12 workouts, here are our top tips for keeping your mojo strong, all the way to the finish line.

Remember why you want this
Re-read your list of motivations from Warm-Up Week to refuel that fire.

Think about how far you've come
Focus on the positives and don't dwell too much on the numbers. Four weeks ago you were only thinking about running, and now you're doing it!

Avoid "all or nothing" thinking
So you missed a workout, you've had a crappy session, or you've found yourself a week behind schedule. This is not a sign from above that "This Running Thing" just wasn't meant to be. You are not doomed to failure. Lace up your shoes and get back out there.

Have fun with your runs
Take a photo of your running locale or your post-run red face and share it on social media. Nag a friend to come with you. Treat yourself to some fancy runner's socks. Shake up the routine with a new running route or run your usual one in reverse.

Think of a post-5k reward
Give yourself something cool to look forward to for when you finish Workout 24: a new book, a magazine subscription, a night out with your friends, or a massage for your hardworking body.

Keep going!
Success is about persistence, not perfection. Think about what a great thing you are doing for yourself. Think about how you want your life to be, beyond the eight weeks of this program. Every step you take is a positive gift to yourself.

Common Running Obstacles

As much as we encourage you to **plan** and execute your 24 workouts in unquestioning robot mode, sometimes you will encounter obstacles that threaten to derail your efforts. But it's **important** to distinguish between a planning challenge and a genuine stumbling block. If you're honest with yourself, deep down you will know the **difference** between a real obstacle and an emotional or time-management issue.

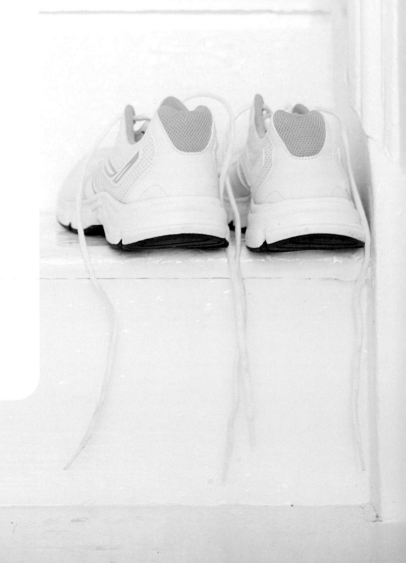

Take emotion out of the equation and look for the solution. How can you adjust and adapt? How can you plan ahead and anticipate challenges? You may need to do things differently from the way you've done them before, but it's only for eight weeks, remember. Let's make it happen!

Here are some common challenges and solutions.

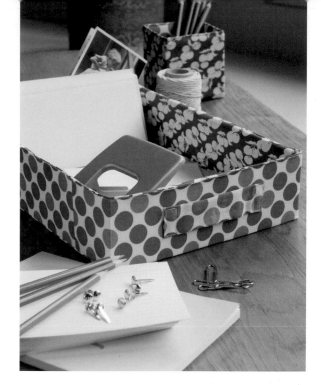

Weather

Rain, hail, heatwaves; Mother Nature loves to throw us a curveball. Look at the weather forecast when you're planning your weekly workouts and choose the best days and times to run. You may need to adjust again on the day of the workout. Look at the challenges of your particular weather and observe your fellow local runners—when do they run? What do they wear? Quite often a workout is just a decent waterproof jacket away.

But if you are having freakish weather and you'd be risking life and limb to run outside, head to the gym and hop on the treadmill—just follow the modifications we've included with each week's training plan.

Don't despair if the weather throws your schedule out a little. If the eight-week program ends up taking you ten, that's okay. You're building the foundation for a lifelong exercise habit. You are in this for the long haul.

Vacation

Going on vacation is no excuse for missing a workout. In fact, it's an even better running scenario. You have fewer things competing for your time and attention, plus it's a fantastic way to explore new surroundings. Find your hotel on Google Maps then "look" around the neighborhood for the nearest park. Search running blogs or forums for popular paths or tracks at your destination. Bring your camera on a morning run and take photos of the local sights before the tourist crowds are awake. Once your run is done, revel in that smugness all day long.

Work

There isn't a job in the world these days that doesn't involve busyness and constantly shifting priorities. Again, anticipation is the key. Look at your schedule and identify the crunch times in your working week. Can you start half an hour earlier and take a longer lunch break to fit in your workout? Many employers are flexible, especially if it improves employee well-being.

If you travel for work, the previous vacation tips will apply. You could also invest in a pair of lightweight running shoes that won't take up much room in carry-on luggage. If socializing and networking is part of your remit, you may need to get up earlier to fit in your run, or tell your colleagues you'll join them just a little later for dinner. Your health is important and you can't beat exercise for shaking off the cobwebs after a long day of sitting in meetings.

Illness

It's important to listen to your body when deciding whether you need to run or rest. Ignoring its signals can hinder your recovery.

If you have a cold that is limited to head symptoms you can try a run—sometimes movement can bring you some relief.

Don't run if:

- You have a fever
- You have a severe cold with chest symptoms
- You have a viral infection
- You're taking antibiotics
- You have any sort of intestinal distress

If any of these apply, rest and let yourself heal. Prescription medicines, especially antibiotics, may need to run their course through your body before you can restart your regular training program. The same advice goes for any sort of intestinal distress. It takes a few days for your body to get back in sync—just remember this when you return to your workouts.

How you resume your training depends on the duration of your illness:

- 1–2 days: pick up from where you left off in the training program.
- 3–7 days: go for a 30-minute walk and try running for a few minutes at a time and see how that feels. If you feel fine afterward, you can resume from where you left off.
- Over seven days: start with a 30-minute walk and then decide if it might be wise to go back one week in the training program. Allowing your body to heal has to be your priority. Err on the side of doing too little rather than too much; there's plenty of time to catch up.

Injury

As we wrote in Week 2, we don't often see severe injuries at the beginning stages of training. If you happen to be one of the unlucky ones with shin fatigue that won't go away or running shoes that keep giving you grief, there are steps you can take to move forward.

- Keep moving. Many people get injured and cease all activity. Usually it's only one part of your body that is injured, so the rest of your body needs to keep active. Replace your three running days per week with another activity that doesn't aggravate your injury, such as swimming, cycling, or gentle walking. If you can keep moving three times a week, you won't have lost all the conditioning when the time comes to restart running.

- Seek help if pain persists. Rather than being an acute injury, sometimes pain is random, sporadic, and will inexplicably disappear with time and rest. But if you're still having issues after two weeks, make an appointment with an osteopath or sports medicine professional.

The halfway point is where you need to dig deep. You are over the shock of the new but the finish line is still a way down the line. Always check in with your motivations from Warm-Up Week if you find yourself flagging. Remember—your runs don't need to be perfect. They just need to be done.

FAQs

Q. Should I run during my period?

A. Running during your period doesn't usually affect your performance. In fact, it can help relieve cramping and ease water retention. Most women can pinpoint a day during their cycle when they feel the most uncomfortable, which tends to be the first or second day after flow begins. Feel free to give yourself a rest day to help your body through the monthly hormonal storm.

When you get back to your running the next day, we recommend you use tampons instead of pads to avoid any chafing.

Week 5 superstar profiles:
Andrea & René Heimes

Age: Both 35
Location: Brüggen, Germany
Occupation:
Andrea — Support Analyst
René — IT Systems Engineer

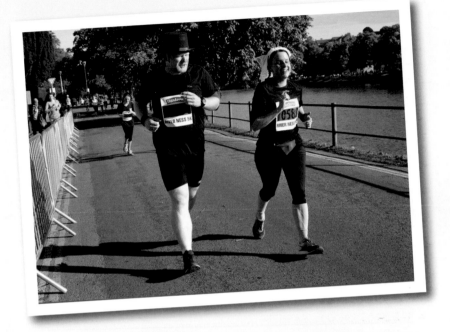

Andrea

I joined a running group at school, but gave up because I always got side stitches. Throughout my twenties I signed up for, and then abandoned, multiple gym memberships.

Then I decided to give running another try, starting with short intervals with walking breaks. Before long, I was running two or three times a week and I bought myself a spot on the Up & Running 10k course. I was nervous because even though I could run a 5k, I hadn't participated in an official race before. But I happily worked through the course without injury and I've gone on to run multiple half marathons.

The longer I've been running, the more people in my life seem to have been infected by the running virus, including my husband René. Having this common interest has really made our relationship even closer. Running together is a great time to relax and talk.

René

I tried several sports but nothing lasted long. Right before I took up running, I was taking the occasional bike ride or playing badminton. However, I was overweight and decided it was time to take up sport more seriously. Plus, Andrea had started running and I wanted to compete with her.

I was off and running as soon as I had a training plan. Running with a plan is always more exciting than just trotting aimlessly around the same path. I look forward to each run and see it as a way to forget the stress of the day. Of course, there are also times when it is hard to motivate myself, but luckily Andrea can help me to get off my behind—and vice versa!

Running is now our shared hobby. We participate in local runs and learn more about our neighboring towns and cities. Our anniversary will be a short trip to Cologne—including running the marathon.

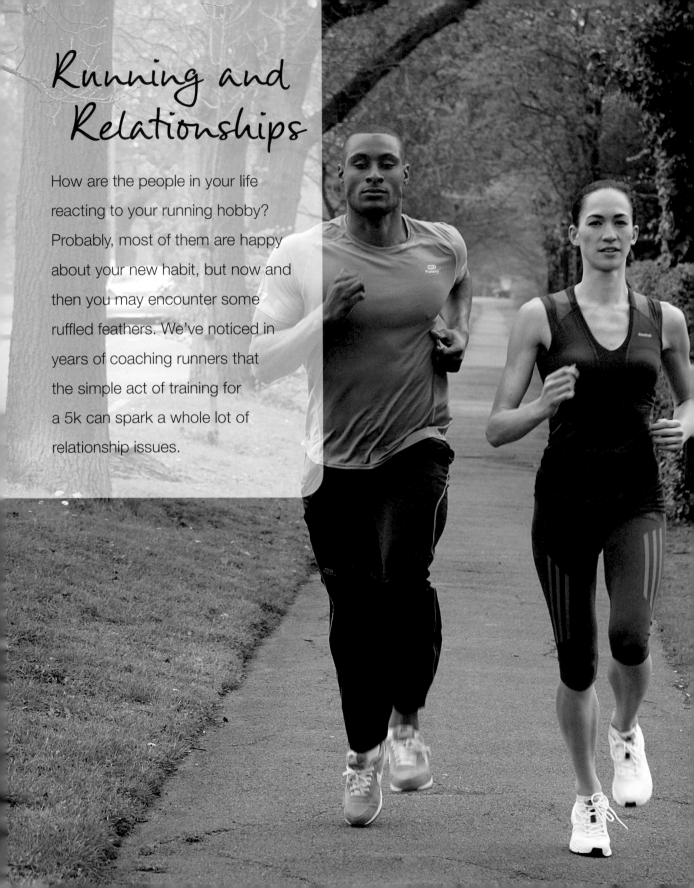

Running and Relationships

How are the people in your life reacting to your running hobby? Probably, most of them are happy about your new habit, but now and then you may encounter some ruffled feathers. We've noticed in years of coaching runners that the simple act of training for a 5k can spark a whole lot of relationship issues.

You may feel that you're simply trotting out for three runs a week, but others may perceive this differently. When a loved one does something new, it can shake the dynamic of a relationship. Whether it's a partner, friend, parent, sibling, colleague, or even your own children, we all establish unwritten rules and boundaries with one another. We have unspoken roles and put comforting routines in place so we behave within a set of boundaries and expectations.

By starting to run, you've challenged the status quo. Some runners meet no resistance—you may have a strong, supportive network of people who are happy that you're making changes. But for many, it's not perceived as a positive thing. A partner feels anxious or envious of your post-run glow if they're still lounging on the couch. A colleague makes snippy comments as you head out for a lunchtime run instead of staying at your desk. Your new hobby can bring deeper insecurities and fears about the relationship to the surface.

You may find it easy to shake off these comments, but if these reactions are challenging your resolve to keep running, here's how to work through them.

- Let your loved ones know how important Project 5k is to you. Explain your motivations to them—share your list from the Warm-Up chapter. If they appreciate the deeper reasons for this project and understand that it's about improving the quality of your life and health, they're more likely to be supportive.
- You may need to do some reassuring that you are the same person and that you're not asking them to change anything about themselves.
- No matter how much you love your running, don't force them to try it, too. Instead, casually invite them to come on a workout with you. If they have no interest in running, they could follow you on a bike to keep you company. It's a great way for couples and friends to spend quality time together.
- Tell them about the positive impact running has already had on your life—that it helps you to be a more cheerful person. Who doesn't want to hang out with a more cheerful person?

My 80-year-old mother always says, 'You'll get hurt, it's bad for your heart, stay home and rest!' I simply don't listen to her. FRANCESCO, ITALY

Everytime I head off to a race, my dad looks at me as if it is the last time he'll ever see me. FIONA, IRELAND

When I started running, my family and friends gave me a lot of support and encouragement. That is, until I signed up for my first race! My friends would comment, "You're crazy! You won't be able to do that!" Or, "That sounds pretty impossible." Now they're used to it and say I was born to run. MICHAEL, USA

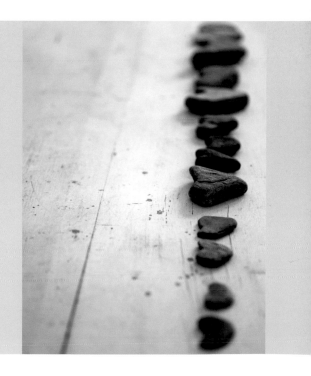

Week 5
Training Plan

- Free Form Walk with arm swings — 5:00
- Stretch — 3:00
- 5 x (5 half squats/10 heel lifts/20 marching steps) — 5:00
- Rest — 2:00
- 3 x (0:5km run/2:00 rest) — 18:00
- 1.5km Free Form Run

Instructions

1 Free Form Walk with arm swings
Warm up with a brisk walk. Swing your arms back and forth, up, and around to get the circulation going.

2 Stretch
Stretch for three minutes now or go straight to the next exercise and leave stretching until the end of your workout.

3 5 x (5 half squats/ 10 heel lifts/ 20 marching steps)
This circuit is done standing in place. Start with five half squats followed by 10 heel lifts. After the tenth heel lift, go straight into your marching steps. Do 10 steps per leg for a total of 20. This circuit has no breaks so after the marching steps start the circuit again with the half squats.

Slow and steady
As you improve your base fitness level and train consistently, your 1km time improvements will be more incremental and you probably won't see the dramatic reductions that have characterized previous weeks. But this is a good thing and shows that you are making progress.

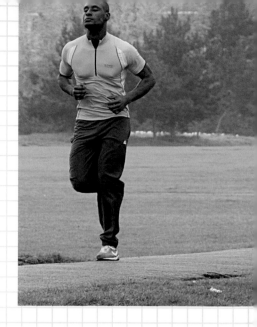

4 Rest
Stretch or walk slowly for two minutes. If you feel ready to continue, skip this rest, and start the next exercise.

5 3 x (0.5km run/ 2:00 rest)
Since you're running 500 meters three times, try to run this exercise a little faster than you would the 1km. You do have a two-minute rest after each run, so really go for it.

6 1km Free Form Run
Give it your best and don't forget to time yourself.

Always improving
Be aware of other great indicators of progress too, such as:
- Feeling energized after a workout rather than completely wiped out
- Stable breathing patterns— no more gasping for breath
- Covering a longer total distance in your workout
- Being able to do more running versus walking during your Free Form Runs

Week 5 Wisdom
The great thing about running in the rain is that there's no one around to witness me marching in place. No, that's not true. The great thing about running in the rain is feeling like I'm better than everyone else who isn't there watching me march in place.
SARA, ITALY

Treadmill Modifications
- For the arm swings, choose a version that allows you to maintain your balance.
- Hop off the treadmill for stretching.
- Stay off the treadmill to perform the half squat/heel lifts/ marching steps sequence.
- For the rest, stretch or Stork next to the treadmill, then hop back on to complete the rest of the workout.

Exercise: Half Squat

The prime targets of this exercise are your gluteus maximus and hamstring muscles, although you may also feel it in your quadriceps.

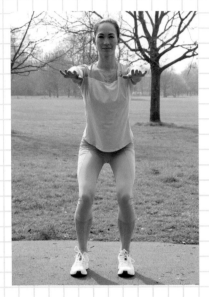

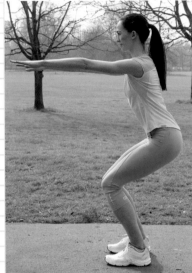

2 Keep your back straight as you bend your knees and go down as far as you can without leaning forward. Come back up by squeezing your glutes and straightening your knees.

1 Stand with feet hip-distance apart and hold your arms out in front for balance.

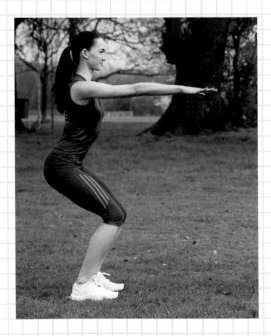

3 Remember, this is a half squat so it's fine if you're only squatting down a few inches.

Tip
Make sure you don't let your knees extend beyond your toes because this puts strain on your knees.

Exercise: March in Place

Use your arms to balance by swinging them back and forth in rhythm as you take your marching steps. Knees can come up as far as you want, even touching your chest. Why march in place? It works your hip flexors, which engage every time you lift your knees. When you run, each of your legs will do this same movement around 80 times per minute, so this group of muscles needs to be strong.

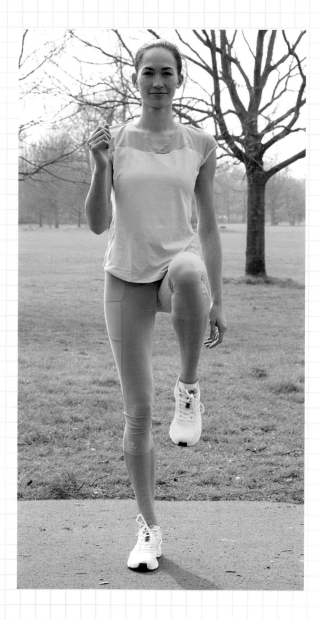
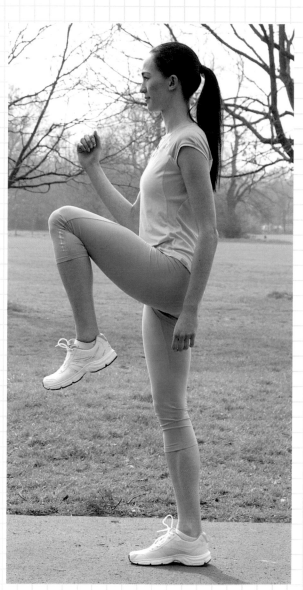

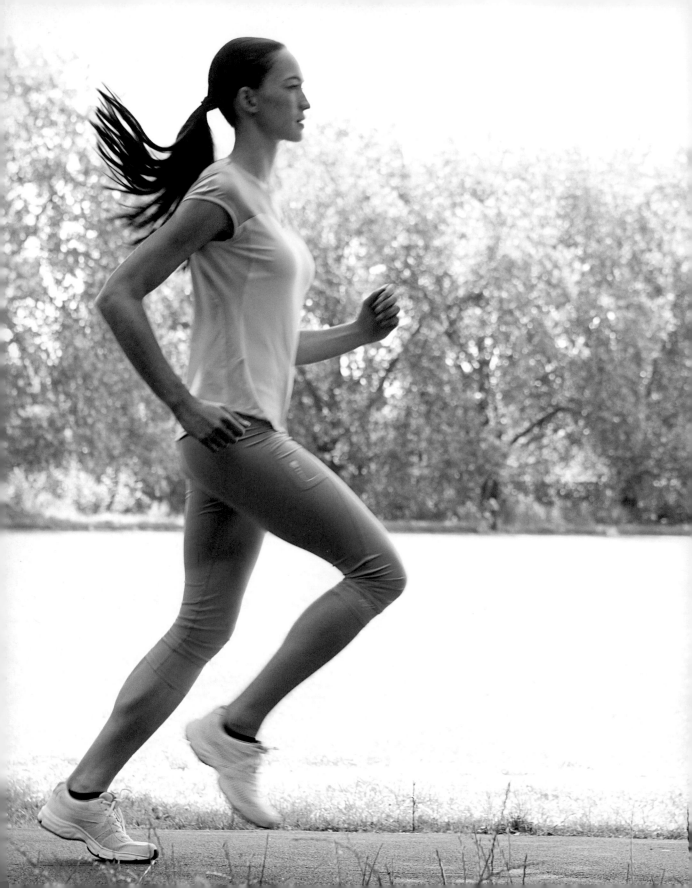

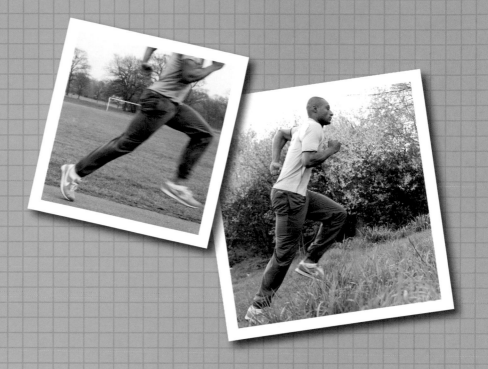

Running Style
and Technique

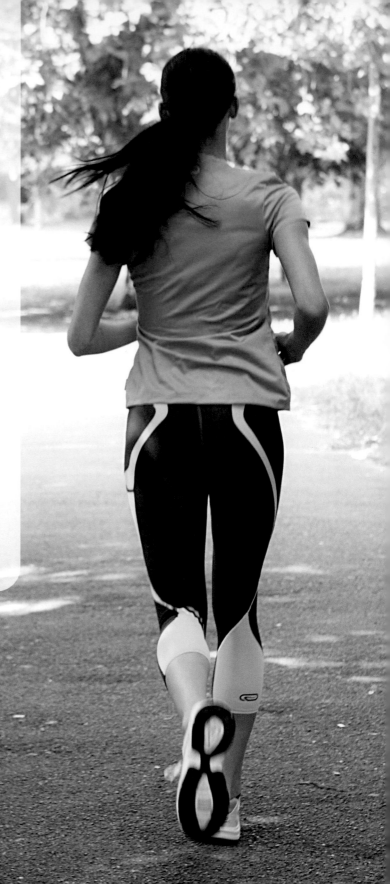

The Right Way to Run

One of the commonest questions we hear from runners is, "What's the right way to run?" You may have heard different **theories** and are wondering whether you should land on your forefoot, mid-sole, or heels. You've noticed that élite athletes or experienced runner friends have a slightly different **running** style from yours. You're convinced that armed with the proper knowledge and advice, you, too, will be on your way to **perfect** running form.

It's a little bit more complicated than that. We all have unique physical characteristics. The way we move and run is influenced by a combination of our genetic makeup, our lifestyle choices, and any mishaps or accidents in the past that may have altered our physiology. Even our mental outlook can affect how our body moves when we run.

Consider how your body moves when you run: your feet and torso, the swing of your arms, your pace and gait. These are all innate and acquired qualities. Have you ever watched British marathon champion Paula Radcliffe run? On every fourth step, her head tilts forward as if she's nodding. The faster she runs, the quicker she nods. During the prime of her career journalists constantly pestered her about this. But she decided that the time and effort it would take to modify her running style would be better spent on training. Despite her "incorrect" running style, she still holds the women's world record for the marathon distance.

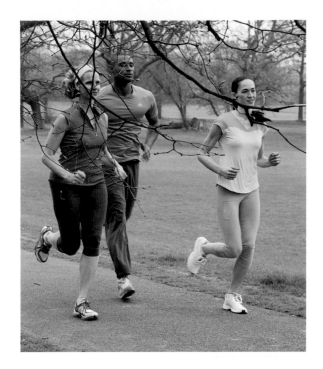

Natural Running Style

So don't worry too much about your running style at this stage of your training. It's more important to build your fitness level and become comfortable running for a few kilometers without too much effort. Once you can run for 30 minutes at what feels like an easy pace, you can start looking at your technique in more depth. In the meantime, here are a few suggestions to help you run with a natural style.

- **Focus your vision straight ahead,** not down at the ground or at your shoes. Enjoy the view or simply gaze at a spot in front of you. If you're constantly looking down, make sure that it's not because you need to run with glasses or contacts.

- **Keep your shoulders relaxed.** Many runners unconsciously tense their shoulders or slump forward while running. Stretch your shoulders before you begin your workout to get them loosened up. Reach your arms above your head, lifting up and then relaxing your shoulders for five or six counts. You can even do this a few times as you run.

- **Keep your elbows loosely bent at a 90-degree angle.** Your arms should be relaxed and move in sync with your legs. Keep your hands relaxed with your fingers slightly closed, not in a tight fist.

- **Pay attention to your feet.** As we explored in the Week 2 chapter, most new runners use their quads while running, putting their weight on the entire foot (from heel to toe), and pushing off from their knees. This takes up a lot of energy and can cause knee injuries. The secret is to use your feet actively. Place your attention on your feet and land on your foot's midsole. Your foot should cushion you and then roll forward, leaving your foot behind. In contrast, landing with your heels breaks your movement and momentum. It can also have traumatic consequences for your back and hips. By focusing on your feet, you'll automatically modify the mechanical action.

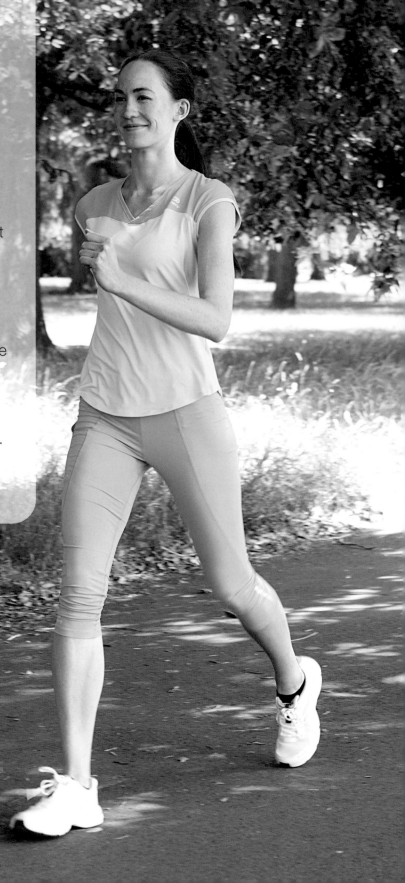

Running versus Walking

One of the most popular goals that new runners have for their first 5k race is to run the entire distance without having to walk. In their desire to become runners, they see walking as a cop-out or failure.

But it's not. Walking can actually be your secret weapon.

In this initial stage of training, it's normal to experience muscular fatigue as your body gets accustomed to new exercises and movement. Walking is the fastest way to restore energy back to those muscles. So don't be afraid to make walking part of your Free Form Runs if you need to do so.

A few short walking breaks can also make you a faster runner. Sound crazy? Take one workout this week to experiment with this simple test. It's easy to do and will give you insight into your running skills.

The Week 6 plan has three 1k Free Form Runs, with a generous three-minute recovery in between. Your experiment is to approach them in three different ways and time each one.

Kilometer 1
Run the entire distance without walking
Start out slowly and keep your breathing controlled. As you feel more comfortable you can increase your speed—or not. The important thing is to run the entire distance without worrying about the final time. If you're not yet up to running the whole kilometer, run as much of it as you can, inserting brief walking breaks.

Kilometer 2
Walk the first 500m and run the remaining 500m
Start out walking at a fast pace until you hit the halfway mark, then run the rest of the way. Remember always to start out slowly, then increase your speed as you progress toward the finish line.

Kilometer 3
Alternate walk 1:00/run 1:00 for the entire 1km
Begin this 1km by walking for one minute, then running for one minute. Alternate this pattern all the way to the end of the distance.

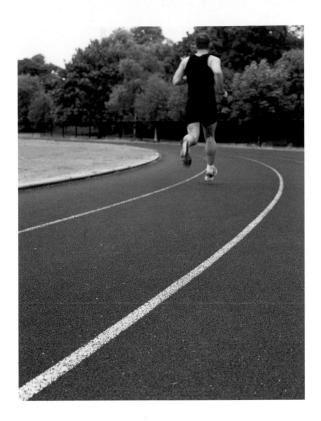

You might be surprised to find that not only are your final times across the three tests quite similar, but that you're actually faster when you have a few walking breaks. If this is the case, we would recommend inserting walking breaks into your training and 5k races. Make sure the walk portion is active and dynamic and not a shame-walk with your head hung down and shoulders collapsing. Continue to use your arms to push you forward. When your breath is under control and the muscle fatigue in your quads or calves dissipates, you can start to run slowly again.

As your body becomes more conditioned and your running style improves, you'll be able to forego the walking breaks. But in the meantime, use them to your advantage.

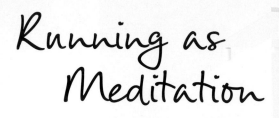

Running as Meditation

The word **meditation** can conjure up images of Buddhist priests sitting gracefully on Himalayan hilltops, eyes closed, in saffron-colored robes. Although true meditation is practiced to reach **heightened** spiritual awareness, the simple exercise of clearing your mind and **concentrating** on one thing at a time can also improve your running.

We live in such a multitasking society that many of us have lost the habit of concentrating on one movement, one activity, one moment. As we begin a workout, myriad thoughts flash across our minds faster than we can keep up with them. Running can help us clear our minds or work through problems—the longer we go on, the more thoughts will thin out and shiny new ideas appear. But running can be hard work if we happen to be in a negative mood—our thoughts can spiral downward pretty fast.

By using meditation techniques when you run, you'll not only clear your mind but also help yourself deal with difficult running moments, whatever the distance. It's a matter of placing your attention on one thought or movement and gently reining in your wandering mind. Here are three running meditation ideas to get you started.

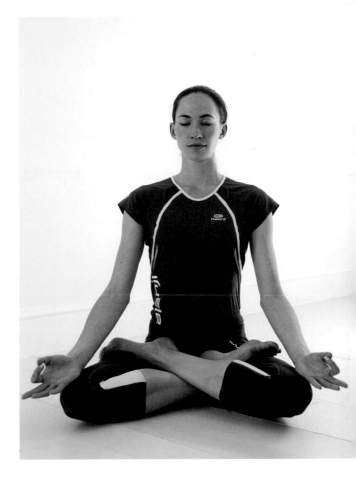

Observe your Breath

Is it easy or labored? Are you taking shallow quick breaths or longer, deeper ones? As you continue to run, take a deep breath and fill your lungs up completely, feeling your belly expand slightly. It doesn't matter whether you take air in through your mouth or nose, either is fine. Purse your lips and exhale, controlling the air as it leaves your lungs. Do this two or three times, then return to your normal breathing pattern. If your breaths are taken in gulps, try decreasing your speed and notice how your breathing pattern changes; or do the opposite and slightly speed up to see if your heart and lungs follow.

Notice the Sound of your Footsteps

Focus on that sound. What do you hear? Do your feet slap down or do you take smaller, dainty steps? Is one foot noisier than the other or do you shuffle as you run? Activate your feet, push off with them, and listen for changes in the sound intensity. If you're running with others, tune into their footsteps and see how they differ from your own.

Dissolve Body Tension

Do a quick mental body scan and notice any areas that feel tense. Start with the muscles in your forehead and jaw. Lift your shoulders up and then drop them to see if there's any tension across your back or in your neck. Drop your arms to your sides for two seconds and then raise them so that with your elbows are at a 90-degree angle. Check to see that your hands are relaxed and not clenched into a tight fist.

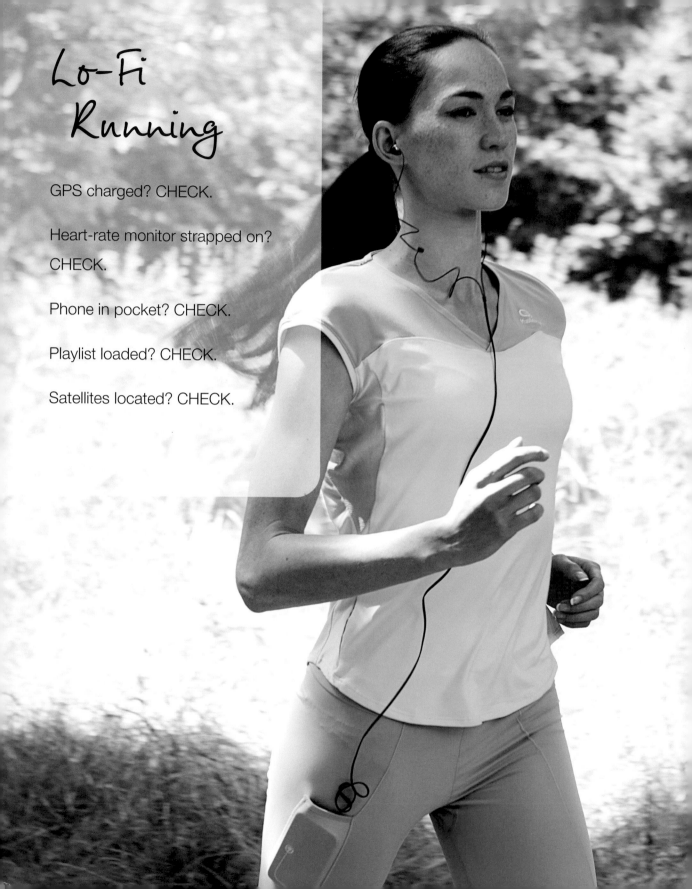

Lo-Fi Running

GPS charged? CHECK.

Heart-rate monitor strapped on? CHECK.

Phone in pocket? CHECK.

Playlist loaded? CHECK.

Satellites located? CHECK.

Congratulations, you are now ready for takeoff! Or is that just the preparation for your 45-minute run?

There are so many running gadgets on offer today that it can feel it takes longer to get ready for your workout than actually to *do* the thing. And once you're finally running, technical hiccups can really disrupt your rhythm—from pressing a wrong button on your running app or losing your satellite connection.

Don't get us wrong: we love gadgetry and wouldn't be without it. We listen to our favorite podcasts and audiobooks while training. But if you find that you have to run with music or you can't run at all, something deeper needs to be addressed.

Now, you don't need to go into therapy, but try running every once in a while without music or audio. This is a particularly good idea if you're planning on running races. Many organizations don't allow you to wear headphones, mainly for safety reasons. But you're also missing out on the atmosphere and camaraderie of the race, which can be far more motivating than the beat of your music.

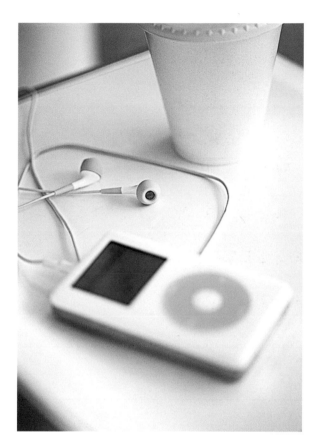

Start with just one headphone-free workout a week. Observe what goes on in your head while you're running. Take a look around at your surroundings. Try to feel comfortable with your own company. Have fun just running.

While you're running, observe what goes on in both your mind and body:

- How's your breathing? Is it shallow or deep?
- What thoughts are popping into your mind?
- How are you arms positioned?
- What do your footsteps sound like? Are you shuffling or actively pushing off the ground?
- How does this running speed feel? Could you pick it up a notch or do you need to take a walking break?
- Now, what's for dinner?

Do gadgets help you when you run?

We asked runners how they use gadgets during their workouts.

I started listening to podcasts during half-marathon training. There's only so much dance and pop you can take for an hour-plus runs, so podcasts are a good way to keep my brain entertained. KATHERINE, UK

I usually run in silence, but often the last song I heard on the radio before heading out will replay in my mind! LUCY, USA

I listened to music when I first started running but now I prefer to listen to my body. MICHELE, ITALY

I prefer to run without music. I like hearing everything happening around me, including my own breathing. I love being able to hear people around me talking during races and exchanging a friendly word or two. JO, AUSTRALIA

I enjoy listening to upbeat music, with only one earphone in. I like to be able to hear other people, cars, dogs, etc—a leftover habit from living and running in West Africa, where I wanted to hear the cars before they got me! JULIA, USA

Music gives me something to concentrate on other than my thoughts. Without it I'd be thinking some negative stuff. Music also provides the tempo for my steps. I love disco hits; the music of my youth! MINNA, FINLAND

Week 6 superstar profile:

Mark Sebastian Stehle

Age: 39
Location: Philadelphia, USA
Occupation: Photographer and musician

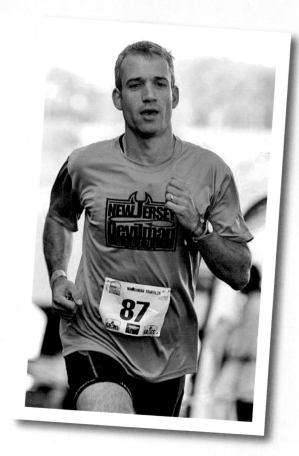

I got involved with running through training for triathlon. My wife is a triathlete, and she introduced me to the sport. My weekly workouts include a minimum of two swims, one run, and one bike workout.

I love the satisfaction of completing a difficult workout and meeting or exceeding my workout goals. It's given me a lot of confidence, which affects all of my athletic pursuits and personal life.

Running reinforced my sense of competitiveness and determination. It is amazing how much my determination to pass the person in front of me or the desire to meet my time-goal affect my ability to run faster, even when I feel I have nothing left.

As a Type I diabetic, running and regular aerobic exercise have brought my blood-sugar levels under amazing control, better than they have ever been in my whole life. If nothing else, this health benefit alone ensures that I make time to fit my workouts into my busy schedule.

Sometimes I have no desire to go out running; then sometimes there is nothing I want more than to go outside and exercise. I have a tendency to succumb to whatever insignificant excuse I can use to skip a workout, especially in the evening after a day at work. But since being given weekly workouts by my wife and signing up for future races, I feel more motivated to overcome those temptations.

Generally, my workouts energize me, even when I have a difficult one involving sprints in high heat and humidity. I usually listen to music, but if there is something on my mind that I need to think through, a quiet run is a great opportunity to do that.

Week 6
Training Plan

- Free Form Walk with arm swings — 5:00
- Slow run — 5:00
- Stretch — 3:00
- 3 x 1km Free Form Run (3:00 recovery in between each)

Instructions

1 Free Form Walk with arm swings
Warm up with a brisk five-minute walk. Swing your arms back and forth, up and around to get the circulation going.

2 Slow run
Break into a slow run for a further five minutes, or you can continue to walk if you prefer.

3 Stretch
No bouncing or jerking moves. Ease into your stretches and get the muscles warmed up.

Recovery time
During your three-minute recovery breaks you can walk, stretch, or meditate.

Week 6 Wisdom
Number of flies that flew into my mouth on my run: 1. Number of flies that I managed to remove from my mouth: 0.5"

PHILIPPA, UK

Treadmill Modifications
- For the arm swings, choose a version that allows you to maintain your balance.
- Do your stretches next to the treadmill or on a mat.

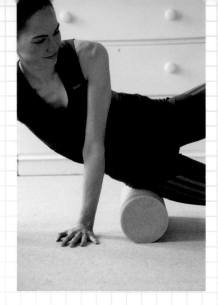

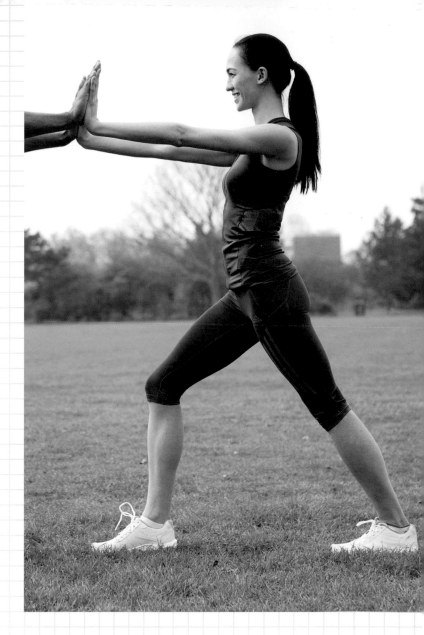

4 3 x 1km Free Form Run (3:00 recovery in between each)

Time each 1km interval and make sure that the first is the slowest. Every once in a while, concentrate on various body parts for a few seconds. Feel your feet and actively push off from the ground in a forward motion. Relax your shoulders and unclench your fists.

Q. Can I run more often?

A. If you feel that your body has adapted to the three weekly workouts and you have energy to burn, feel free to add a fourth run. This can boost your progress by about 20 percent. That's a big leap for an extra 45 minutes.

At this stage of your training, we don't advise running more than four days per week. Just make sure you're supporting your activity with nutritious meals and plenty of sleep. The combination of the two will help you recover and be ready for your next run.

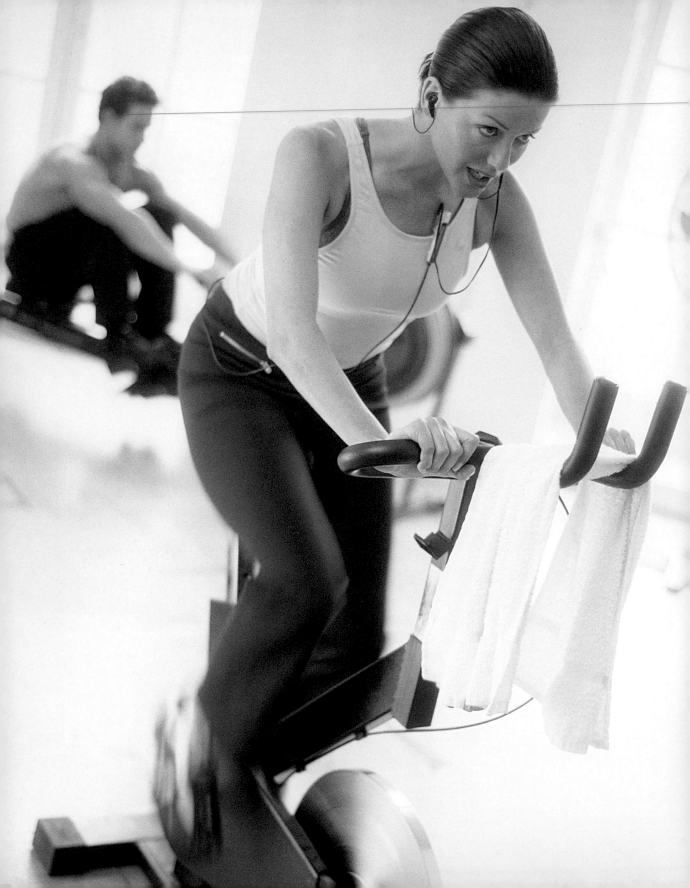

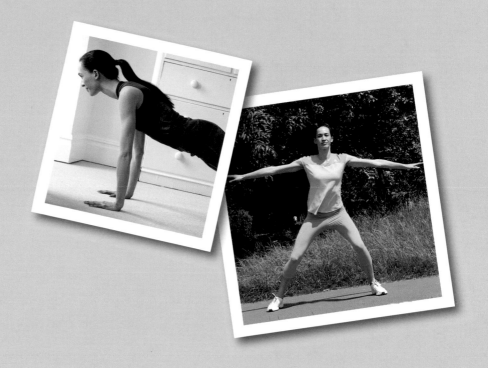

Cross Training

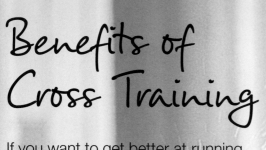

Benefits of Cross Training

If you want to get better at running you need to run. But always keep in mind that running is a high impact sport. If your body isn't well conditioned, those endorphin highs can come at a price. That's where cross training steps in.

Cross training has a very simple definition: any sports activity other than the one for which you predominately train. Cycling, swimming, yoga, badminton, you name the sport—that is cross training to your main running activity.

Once you go beyond this 5k program and integrate running fully into your everyday life, we recommend adding regular cross training to your schedule. It can have fantastic benefits for your running.

■ It adds variety to your workouts and improves overall fitness. No matter how much you love running, you might feel the need for a mental break once in a while. Getting in the pool or hopping on a bike mixes things up. Choosing a team sport can be a nice contrast to the solitary nature of running.

■ It helps prevent injury. Adding a cross-training workout to your week will stimulate muscles that normally don't get used while you run. It also gives the overworked muscles an "active" rest from your normal routine.

■ You'll maintain your conditioning if you do get injured. When a medical professional tells you to rest while injured, they don't mean sitting on the couch watching television. They mean active rest. Cross training with an activity that doesn't aggravate your injury, such as swimming, can keep you aerobically fit and maintained while you heal. Many athletes have actually found themselves running stronger and faster after an injury.

■ It balances out your muscle groups. You predominantly use your leg muscles while running, rarely the upper half of your body. Over time this can create an imbalance between your lower and upper body strength. By choosing a cross-training activity that works your arms, you'll develop upper-body strength that's impossible to achieve with running alone. Plus, a balanced body will function better and look aesthetically more pleasing.

Start with just one cross-training session per week. Aim for consistency rather than setting up a crazy, unsustainable training schedule. And remember, your main goal is to run a 5k, so make sure you get those three runs in before adding any other activity.

Anything goes for cross training, although you may want to try a sport that will complement your running, such as:

■ Outdoor cycling or indoor spinning
■ Swimming
■ Rowing
■ In-line or roller-skating
■ CrossFit or plyometrics
■ Zumba or other dance classes
■ Yoga or Pilates

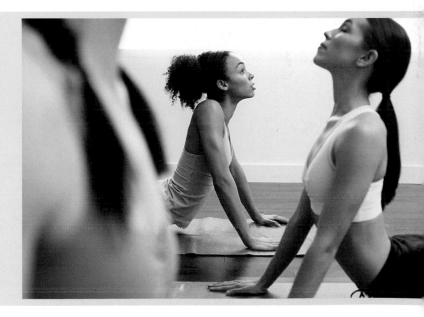

How does cross training help your running?

From hiking to cycling, yoga to rock climbing, the possibilities are almost endless when it comes to choosing a cross-training activity. We asked some runners to tell us about their cross-training routines and how their running benefits from them.

I like cycling for cross training, especially cycle touring as it involves lots of coffee, scones, and jam and cream!
PAUL, UNITED ARAB EMIRATES

Once a week, I go on a one-hour hike with a close friend. It's fun to catch up on each other's news and admire the birds and vistas and nature in general. Even when the weather is not ideal we go out anyway. We have been caught out on a ridge in high winds, bracing each other so the wind wouldn't knock us down. We've been in snow so thick we weren't sure we were heading the right way back to the car. We've logged a lot of hours over the last three years, and I know I would have found excuses to miss if she wasn't looking forward to our day! CASSIDY, USA

I love rock climbing. It's not just the upper-body work you think it's going to be. It's a fantastic workout for body and brain. TOR, UK

I play basketball once a week. Before I started running, I was completely drained after 20 minutes of play. Now that I'm training for my first ultra marathon, I can finish a game without breaking a sweat.
ALESSANDRO, ITALY

I like yoga as it promotes focus on what your body can achieve in that moment. This translates well into running. The balancing and stretching are complementary to running. I also like boxing. I enjoy the upper-body workout and the sound my glove makes when it hits the bag. JULIA, USA

Week 7 superstar profile: Alexandra Merrett

Age: 39
Location: Melbourne, Australia
Occupation: Lawyer

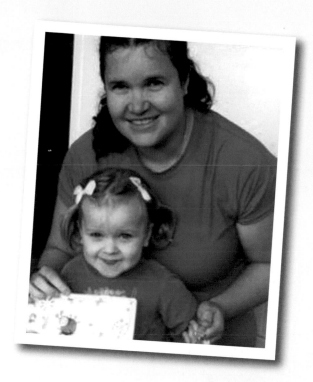

I was active in team sports in high school and university. But exercise took a big hit when I started working horrible hours at a major law firm, although I virtuously kept paying my gym membership and sometimes I even showed up.

I took up running after a winter of illness (asthma and bronchitis). Clearly I needed to exercise, but it had to be super flexible in order to fit around work and the changing sleep schedule of my young daughter. Running was an efficient option that also enabled me to exercise my frisky dog.

I ran on chilly mornings at 5:30am, squeezing in a workout before the childcare/work run. I'd put the baby in a stroller, tether the dog to it, and away we'd all go! I've learned that if I don't run in the morning, I generally don't run. So I get my clothes out the night before, go to bed early, and then leave the house before I've had time to talk myself out of it. If I fail to do any of those things, my chances of getting out fall drastically.

You can't beat the post-run satisfaction of actually having done something—I carry it with me the whole day. And so long as I haven't pushed myself too hard, there's a perverse pleasure in the "good kind of hurt" that is the DOMS (Delayed Onset of Muscle Soreness).

It's been fun to get obsessed by something I'm really not very good at. That said, I'm very young in my running career and have a lot of room for improvement, and I love that.

On a different note, I always try to run when I'm traveling and I've run in some very cool places. Running along the lake in Queenstown, New Zealand is one of many highlights.

Week 7 Exercise
The Plank

Want a simple, portable, and powerful introduction to cross training that you can start right now? Let us introduce you to the plank.

We love the plank because it's a great all-in-one conditioning exercise. It strengthens and stabilizes the muscles in your shoulders, abdomen, and hips. You can do it at home after your workouts or any time during the day when you want to add in some extra movement. It's easy to learn and can be adapted to any fitness level.

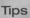

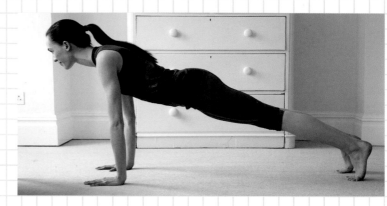

Start out by getting on the floor on all fours. Keep your arms straight and directly beneath your shoulders and extend your legs straight behind you, maintaining your balance on the balls of your feet. You should look as if you were going to do a push-up.

Tips

- Imagine your whole body forming a straight line as you engage your abdominal muscles by tilting your pelvis and pulling your belly button toward your spine.
- Squeezing your glutes will also help you engage your core muscles and maintain the pose for longer.
- Make sure that your weight is distributed evenly between your arms and legs while you concentrate on keeping your back as straight as a wooden plank (hence the name).
- If you're new to planking, start out with just 30 seconds per session, three or four times per week. As you improve your technique, you can increase your time up to five full minutes.

Advanced version

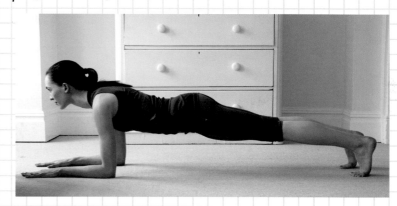

Instead of keeping your arms straight, bend your elbows and rest your body weight on your forearms.

Week 7
Training Plan

- Free Form Walk with arm swings — 5:00
- Slow run — 5:00
- 2 x (10 side skips right/10 side skips left/20 marching steps in place/1:00 slow walk/2:00 fast walk) — 8:00
- 2km Free Form Run
- Rest — 5:00
- 1km Free Form Run

Instructions

1 Free Form Walk with arm swings
Warm up with a brisk walk. Swing your arms back and forth, up and around to get the circulation going.

Think positive
Don't underestimate your capability. Try running a little longer or faster during the running segments.

2 Slow run
Break into a slow run for a further five minutes, or you can continue to walk if you prefer.

3 2 x (10 side skips right/ 10 side skips left/ 20 marching steps in place/1:00 slow walk/ 2:00 fast walk)
Turn sideways. Begin by stepping sideways to the right with your right leg. Take a small "hop" and close the gap with your left leg. Repeat 10 times. Now go back the other way for 10 skips, starting by stepping sideways with your left leg. While you do this exercise, notice that most of the work is being done with your feet and ankles, which are your real target. Now do 20 marching steps in place, that's 10 per leg. Lift your knees as high as possible. Follow this with a minute of slow walking and then two minutes of fast walking. Repeat the whole sequence (see page 119 for step-by-step photographs for this exercise).

4 2km Free Form Run
Run, walk, or do a mix of both in whatever proportions you want, steady and slow.

5 Rest
Take a full five minutes of easy walking or simple stretching before the next segment.

6 1km Free Form Running
Since this is the last segment, try pushing yourself a little more than you did during the 2km run. Remember to record your times.

Focus on finishing
For your first 5k race (real or virtual), your goal is simply to finish. After that you can start looking at a stopwatch and setting yourself time-based goals.

Week 7 Wisdom
Even though today's run wasn't my best experience, I know it's just a single run of the hundreds I'll do. If I keep going, my body will figure it out. All I need to do is to show up.

SARA, ITALY

Treadmill Modifications
■ For the arm swings, choose a version that allows you to maintain your balance.
■ Hop off the treadmill for stretching.
■ Do the side skip/marching sequence off the treadmill. Find a space to do the side skips. You can do them in groups of five if you have a small space. Hop back on the treadmill for the walking segments.

Running Drills

Some Up & Runners refer to them as those "crazy exercises," but the exercises you've been doing throughout the program have an official name: running drills.

Running drills are exercises designed to improve your running form. They help strengthen muscle groups used for running, especially those in your feet, legs, and hips. Practicing drills regularly will train your body to incorporate those same movements into your own running style.

Many runners squirm when they see drills on their training plan. "I just want to run!" they protest. But if you want to improve your running style and avoid injury, you need to do more than just run. The best way to welcome drills into your running routine is by understanding their purpose. Marching in place forces you to lift your knees and activate your glutes and hamstrings. Skipping (everybody's favorite!) strengthens your feet and, if you're a shuffler, teaches you to push off the ground with your feet.

If you feel self-conscious about doing drills, just remember that every professional runner includes them in his or her training program. You're training like the best!

Week 7 **Exercise**
Side Skips

Here's the final drill of the 5k program. Side skips are a basic foot-agility exercise. Notice that most of the work is being done by your feet and ankles because that's the area you're targeting.

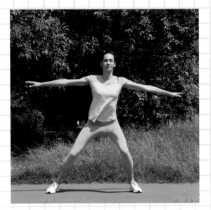

1 Turn sideways and step sideways to the right with your right leg.

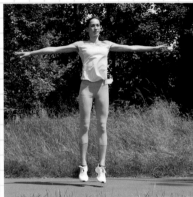

2 Take a small "hop" and close the gap with your left leg.

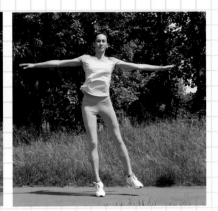

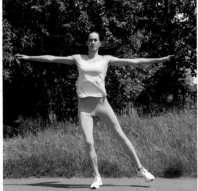

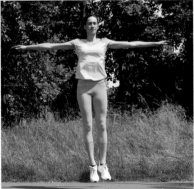

3 Repeat 10 times. Now go back the other way for 10 skips, starting by stepping sideways with your left leg.

Tip
You don't need to come up high as you skip. Keeping your feet low to the ground is fine.

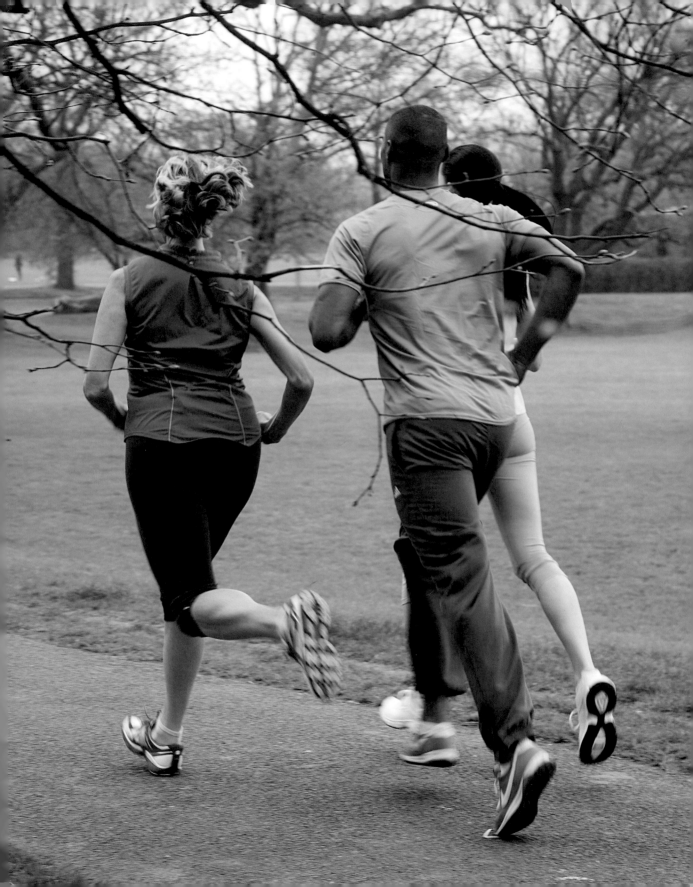

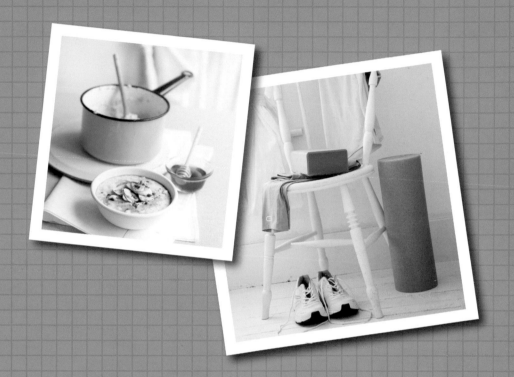

Race Time

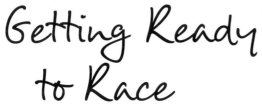

Getting Ready to Race

Here you are at Week 8 with **23 workouts** ticked off and just one more to go—the race. It may not have been easy to prepare your body and mind for this event over the past eight weeks. But if you've been diligent and done all the workouts, trust us, your race will be an **experience** to enjoy.

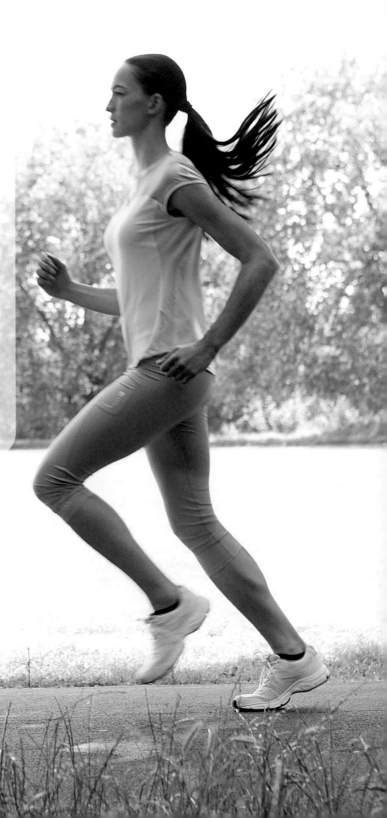

We want your 5k event to be more than just about your finishing time. Whether you've signed up for a small local charity race or a big-city bash with thousands of runners, be sure to make this a special day.

Invite friends and family to run with you or to be your cheer squad. Hold a celebratory pre- or post-race gathering. Your race is the icing on the cake, the treat for all your hard training. Make it a positive one in any way you can.

The key to a great race day is a well-laid plan. You won't be as nervous if you feel in control and know the steps you need to take from the start to finish line. If you have experience with other types of races, you'll know the drill and can personalize your pre- and post-race rituals. If you're new to racing here's our blueprint for success.

The Week Leading Up to the Race

- Study the race course. It could be an out and back route through a city center or a loop through a park, but the most important thing to look for is elevation changes. If you know where the hills are you can plan your race strategy accordingly.
- Check the race day weather forecast. Knowing if you're in for rain or shine will help you decide how to dress. Many runners make the mistake of overdressing and end up overheating during the race. Remember that your 5k could take you anywhere from 20 to 50 minutes to complete, so keep things simple:
- Cold weather: Add fleece gloves, a headband that covers your ears or a thermal hat, ankle-length running pants, long sleeve shirt, and a light windbreaker jacket.
- Hot weather: Sunscreen, running cap, sunglasses, tank top, shorter running pants.

Before your Race

The 5k distance is relatively short, so there's no need for special pre-race nutrition or "carbo-loading." That won't come into play until you're running longer distances. As long as your everyday meals follow the guidelines we gave you in Week 4 and you're eating a variety of foods, you'll be good to go on race day.

The Night Before—Get Your Bag Ready

Being organized will calm your nerves and ensure you don't forget anything. Avoid doing this at the last minute when nerves have already taken hold.

Here's our packing list:
- Bib number or copy of registration if you still need to pick one up at the race
- Safety pins to pin the bib to your shirt
- Watch, heart-rate monitor or GPS
- A change of clothes for after the race
- Sunglasses
- Wipes, travel soap, towel
- Sunscreen
- Hair items for long hair: bands, pins
- Tissues or extra toilet paper (those porta potties often run out...)
- A little cash for a post-race treat

Well-organized races will have a bag-deposit area so you can safely store your gear while you run.

- For morning races, eat a breakfast with complex carbohydrates, such as whole-grain bread or oatmeal, and allow a couple of hours for digestion. For afternoon races, have a light early lunch and include some pasta or rice. At the end of your meal you should feel full but not stuffed.

- Avoid foods that might irritate your stomach or intestinal tract while racing. During your training you probably identified the foods you don't get along with, for example coffee or dairy products. Since you already drink plenty of water during the day and your nutrition plan is packed with fresh fruits and vegetables, you don't need to "fill up" pre-race. Drink according to thirst and stop drinking at least a half hour before your start time, otherwise you'll waste time in bathroom lines.

- Don't worry if you find yourself making several trips to the restroom before your race. It's your autonomic nervous system working at its best. The sympathetic nervous system, which is a component of the autonomic nervous system, will (among other things) constrict your blood vessels, causing you to urinate more often. The parasympathetic nervous system, another component, will increase intestinal activity. Just make sure you find the bathrooms and check the length of the lines so you can estimate how long a visit will take. This may take more planning than your actual race.

At the Start Line

- Do a 10-minute warm up shortly before heading for the start line. Try a fast walk, total body stretch, and even a few skips to get your feet activated. Running for a few minutes might help relieve some of the pre-race tension.
- Most 5k races have a mass start. Many first-time racers underestimate themselves and line up at the very back of the crowd. Choose a spot somewhere in the middle. If you're in the front with the pro runners, you risk getting mowed over or swept away in the excitement and going out too fast. If you line up at the back of the pack, you'll find yourself fighting through the crowds of walkers, strollers, and groups.

Running your Race

You're ready to go, the music is blasting over the speakers, and you feel the adrenaline running through your veins. This is the trickiest part of the race because when they fire that starting gun you need to be in total control and begin by…running slowly. Going out too fast is the number-one mistake that runners make, whether running a 5k or a marathon. It will be tempting to rush. Everybody around you will be going wild, running as fast as they can to get ahead of the crowd. You could be tricked into feeling like this is your special day to be super fast.

The easiest way to take command of your race is to have a plan. So what's yours going to be?

- **Run the whole race.** Take a look at your average 1km times over the past few weeks of training and decide your 5k target time. The most important element is not to go under your average time in the first kilometer of the race. Once the crowds have thinned out and you have more space to run, get your breathing under control. At that point decide if you want to speed up a little or simply cruise along to the finish.
- **Mix walking and running.** There is no shame in walking, especially when it's part of your plan. The key is to decide ahead of time how often and how long your walking breaks will be. For a 5k race we suggest a one-minute walk for every 1km, starting with the walk. If you have the first minute to get settled into the race, you'll be running through the finish line. During your walk segments, concentrate on getting control of your breath and keeping a nice pace. You can also stretch your arms above your head to relieve any tension in shoulders and arms.

During your 5k Race

- A lot of events offer food on the course but for a 5k you won't need to refuel. You have all the energy you need. Take a sip of water at an aid station if you like.
- Use other runners to help you get to the finish line. Pick someone out ahead of you (bright-colored shirts are the easiest) and concentrate on slowly gaining on that person—then pass. It not only helps pass the time but it can be a great psychological boost.
- Whether you decide to walk or run up hills, how you approach them is the same: slow down slightly, shorten your stride length, get into a rhythm, and use your arms to push up to the top.
- Finish the race strong, even if it's just the last 100 meters. It's always a positive feeling to give your best at the end of the race, and you'll take that with you in the weeks after your event.

After your Race

- Celebrate like crazy. No "coulda, shoulda, wouldas!" Let the joy sink in that you have accomplished what you set out to do. Training for, then running, a race is a huge achievement and you deserve to feel great about that.
- After you cross the finish line, take a few minutes to walk around and let your heart recover and breathing return to normal. You can do a few gentle stretches if you wish.
- Now is the time to get something to drink and if you feel like treating yourself to something special, go ahead. Just remember that there's no need to "refuel" for the 5k distance. Don't go overboard!
- Find your bag with your fresh change of clothes and get out of your sweaty race clothes as soon as you can. You'll feel better and have less of a chance of getting cold when you stop moving around.

Create your Own 5k Race

If you can't find an official race that's convenient or near you, you can create your own along with family and friends. No matter where you run, consider it "The" event.

- Decide when and where to do your 5k. It could be at your local track or on a familiar training route that you've already measured out. Give it a specific time and date to make it official.
- Make your course a loop so you'll start and finish at the same point. Your friends can cheer you on as you start out, then celebrate with you at the finish line.
- Invite a seasoned runner to keep you company and pace you.

Racing Jitters Debunked

- **I'm going to be last.** This common fear rarely materializes, but where you end up in the results list depends on the competition. Try to choose events with fun themes or that are run for charity rather than 5,000 meters around a track. That way there's a slimmer possibility of you coming in as organizers dismantle the race course. Another trick is to look at the previous year's results online and check the time of the last runner to get an idea of the field.

- **I won't look like a runner.** Runners come in all shapes, sizes, and ages. Most don't look like the ones in running magazines. They won't have had the advantage of perfect lighting and airbrushing-skills. You'll be surprised at the diversity of runners' bodies at your race, and sometimes people who don't "look" like runners turn out to be the ones having the most fun.
- **I'll be disappointed by my time.** This is your first 5k race. Your main objective is to complete it and get a time for the 5km distance on which you can then build. When you analyze your final time, take your emotions out of the equation. Look at the numbers as what they are—just numbers. They are not a reflection of your self-worth; they're simply a base time that will help you decide what your next step will be. And since this is your first race, any result will mean a personal best!

Post-Race Analysis

We hope you're savoring your post-race runner's high. That is how a race is supposed to feel like—not a struggle, but a reward for all the work you did to get to the starting line.

As you admire your shiny medal, you may be replaying those five kilometers in your head and wondering whether you could have done things differently. Don't analyze your 5k too much. Just note things that you'd like to improve upon next time:

- Did you over- or underdress?
- Did you position yourself correctly at the start?
- Did you go out too fast?
- Could you have pushed yourself a little faster or did you feel you ran well in a comfort zone?

The more you race, the more comfortable you'll feel in the race atmosphere and the easier it will get. Now go and sign up for the next one!

What are your race rituals?

Most runners, from top athletes to those running their first 5k, have a few little rituals to help them prepare for race day. We asked some Up & Runners to share their race rituals.

I have a ritual of pinning my race number to my shirt the night before and writing inspirational notes to myself on it. ANDRE, ITALY

Pre-race ritual: try not to cr*p myself from nerves. Post-race ritual: try not to die and/or throw up from exhaustion! HELEN, UK

I spread out my running clothes on the bed, pin my race number to my shirt, then ask myself, 'what the hell am I doing?' JED, USA

My favorite thing about races is the people. I like eavesdropping on conversations, seeing the diversity of the runners, admiring the outfits. I love interacting with the spectators. I also like telling myself that I'm happy to be there and 'Isn't this all great?!' Basically, for me, it's time to go very Pollyanna. CELIA, BELGIUM

If I'm driving to a race, I have a playlist blaring on the way. I don't run with music, but in the car it makes me smile and (sort of) believe that I'm feeling excited rather than anxious. JO, AUSTRALIA

I always participate in the group warm-up at races, even if it feels a bit stupid. It somehow creates the atmosphere that we are all in this together. MINNA, FINLAND

Week 8 superstar profile: Anne Taylor

Age: 50
Location: Australia
Occupation: Architect

Signing up for Up & Running was an impulsive and uncharacteristic decision. For 20 years I'd been a swimmer, but my access to pools became limited and I wanted something new. I never considered I'd run more than five kilometers, if I even managed to run that.

At first I was self-conscious about wearing "proper" running gear—as if I wasn't entitled. I started out in old T-shirts and leggings with a pair of cheap and nasty shorts over the top. I let myself buy nicer gear as it became clear that I wasn't giving up, that it was more than just a phase.

I learned to trust Coach Julia. That was the critical element in moving beyond 5km. Once I'd established that absolute trust I didn't have to doubt my ability—I just had to do the training. I learned that if I could do five kilometers, then ten were possible, because previously I thought I could run exactly zero kilometers. If you keep doubling the distance, you get to a marathon eventually.

I hardly ever want to go running. Often the runs I dread the most are fine, and the ones I think will be fine are really hard. I think this unknown contributes to my reluctance. I try to tell myself that I choose to do this. Or, I try not to think at all and just go.

I go through the whole range of emotions, from sublime and ecstatic through to disgust with myself for even believing this is possible. I listen to my music, often to music from different periods in my life or music I've just been to see live. Sometimes I have revelations, usually about how to look at things differently so I can move on from something that's been bothering or upsetting me.

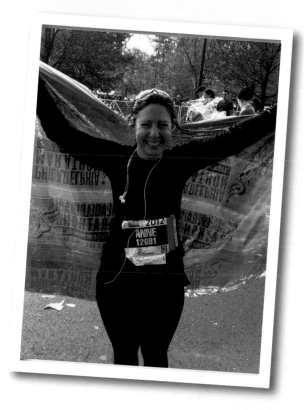

My most memorable running moment was at the start of the Melbourne marathon, my second marathon. I was nervous, but not because I didn't think I could finish. I had no doubt I'd finish. I was nervous that I was about to undertake something that would be really hard and probably hurt. Knowing that I'm not nervous about the distance of a marathon was a beautiful realization.

If I could go back in time and give advice to Anne the beginner, I would tell her nothing. The best bit has been the slow unfolding of running in my life.

Week 8
Training Plan

- Free Form Walk with arm swings — 5:00
- Slow run — 5:00
- Stretch — 3:00
- 2km Free Form Run
- Rest — 5:00
- 2 x 1km Free Form Run (3:00 recovery in between)

Instructions

1 Free Form Walk with arm swings
Warm up with a brisk walk. Swing your arms back and forth, up and around to get the circulation going.

2 Slow run
Break into a slow run for a further five minutes, or you can continue to walk if you prefer.

3 Stretch
Take three minutes to stop for a good stretch.

Double workout
This workout is to be done twice this week. Your third workout is your 5k race!

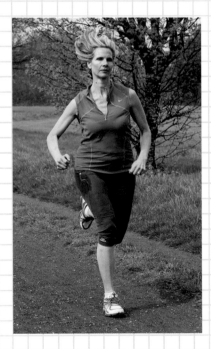

Mix it up
Vary your speed by picking it up a bit toward the end of the running segments.

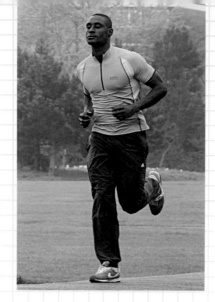

4 **2km Free Form Run**
Run, walk, or do a mix of both in whatever proportions you want. Keep it steady and slow.

5 **Rest**
Take a full five minutes of easy walking or simple stretching before the next segment.

6 **2 x 1km Free Form Run (3:00 recovery in between)**
You'll be running 1km twice with a three-minute rest in between. Free Form Run the first 1km slower than the second. Give the second 1km your very best effort.

Week 8 Wisdom
I want to jump up and down, spin, yell, cry. I've gone from barely being able to run down the street to running 5km. These eight weeks were just the first steps into something amazing.
AMANDA, USA

Treadmill Modifications
■ For the arm swings, choose a version that allows you to maintain your balance.
■ Hop off the treadmill for stretching.

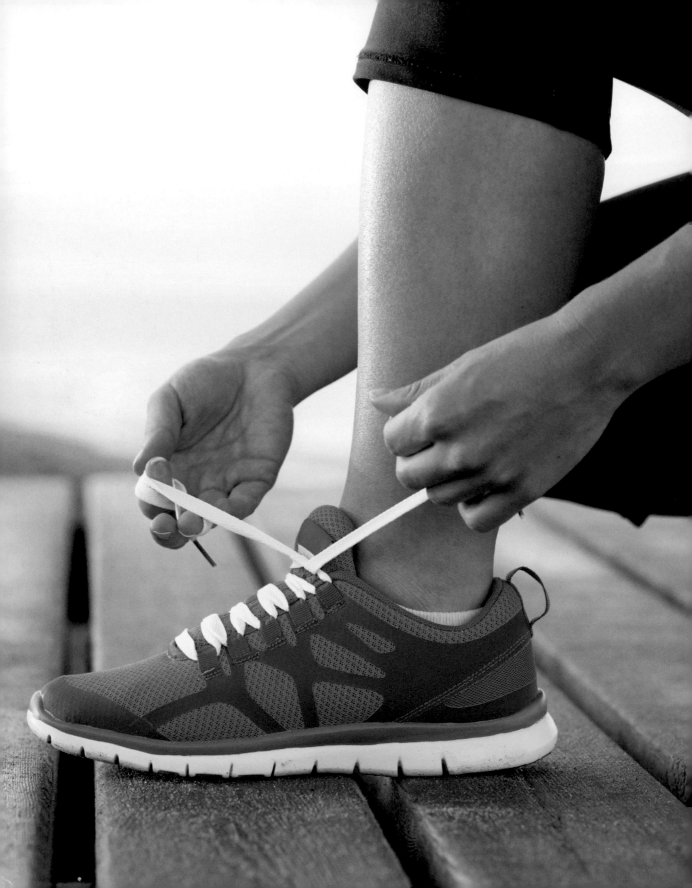

Beyond the 5k

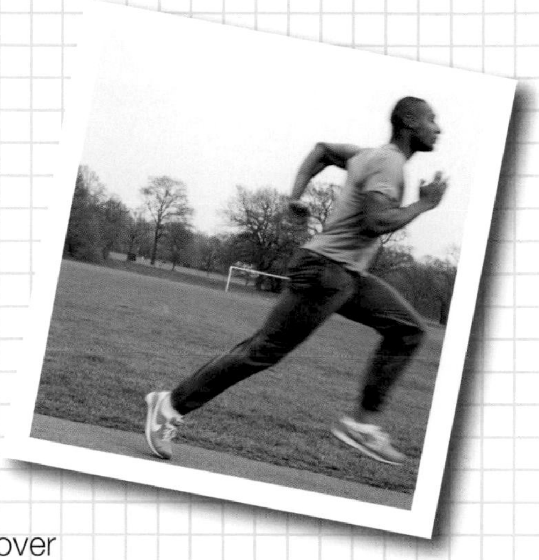

Now that you've ticked off your first 5k race what's the next logical step? Many runners immediately think, "On to the 10k!" But that's not always the best option, at least not right away. The first question to ask is "What are you ready for?"

We want you to enjoy running and love the sport. We want you to avoid injury and build a solid base of fitness that evolves over time. We want you to grow into the various distances, from 5k to 10k and beyond.

So, we have a guideline: **In order to train for a 10k, you should be able to run 5k in 35:00 or under.**

If it takes longer than 35 minutes, it's because you need to work on one or more of the following:

- Your aerobic base
- Your running style
- Your body composition

No matter where you are right now, we have the perfect plan to help you move beyond the 5k and become a stronger, fitter runner.

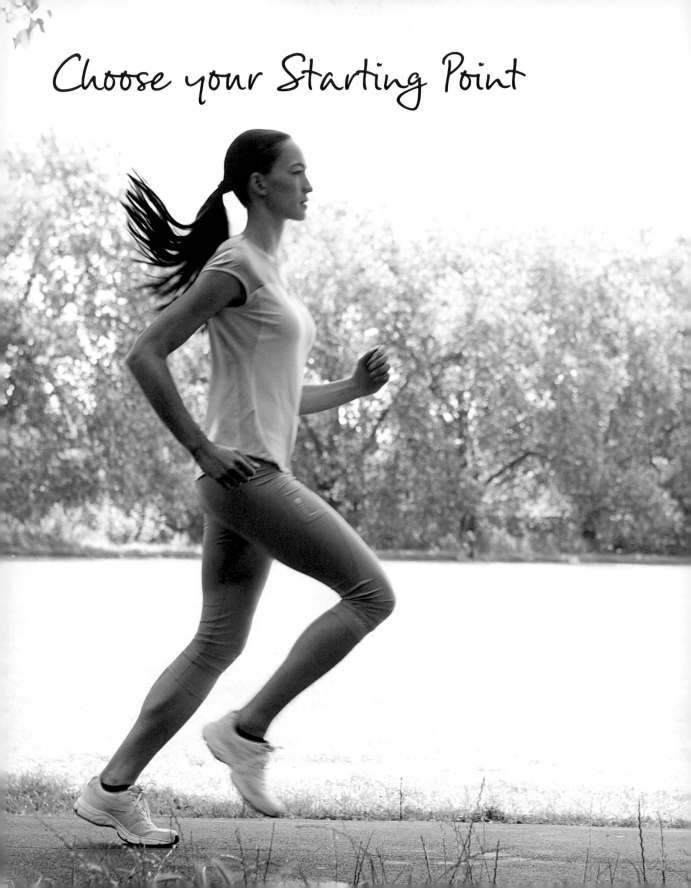

Choose your Starting Point

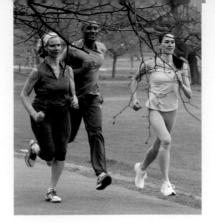

1 If your 5k race time was over 45:00

The best option to improve your running is to repeat the 5k program, skipping Week 1 and beginning from Week 2. If you were diligent about recording your training data over the past eight weeks, you'll be able to compare your times from the first and second rounds and note your improvements.

2 If your 5k race time was between 35:00 and 45:00

You're in the perfect position to tackle any of the "Beyond the 5k" training plans in this chapter. They'll all help you improve your 5k race time. Choose the plan that addresses your running concerns, or just pick the one that looks the most interesting to you. Getting faster is only a matter of accumulated running mileage, so train consistently and be patient.

3 If your 5k race time was under 35:00

Use the "Beyond the 5k" training plans to get your body in peak condition and start thinking about the 10k. All three plans will improve your endurance, stamina, and strength. Mix and match workouts or simply belt out a 5k workout run for fun. Sign up for more races and look for in-between distance events, such as 4 miles or 8k, using any of the "Beyond the 5k" plans to get you race ready.

Bonus boost

No matter what your 5k time, you can give your training an extra boost by adding a fourth workout each week. This can be a simple 40-minute Free Form Run or any other aerobic-based exercise, such as cycling, swimming, or fast walking. This will improve your general conditioning by around 20 percent and also aid in fat loss, if that happens to be on your wish list.

How to Keep the Momentum

It's common to feel slightly lost after the triumph of your first race. For eight long weeks you were focused on reaching your 5k goal. Without that dangling carrot, your motivation can falter and your shiny new exercise habit can start to look a little wobbly.

How do you stop that fire from fizzling out? You need a new plan.

If you simply say, "I'll run a few times a week," your efforts can drift. We encourage you to follow the formula of the past eight weeks: have a plan, know your motivations, and set tangible goals. This holy trinity will keep your fitness habit humming along.

Here's how to replenish your running mojo for life beyond the 5k:

1 Choose your running plan
Check out the following plans and the recommendations at the beginning of this chapter and decide how you'll structure your training.

2 Refresh your motivation
You've come a long way since you made your list in Warm-Up Week. Your initial reasons for wanting to run may not speak to you as strongly today. What's going to inspire you now? Regularly check-in with why you're doing this.

3 Set new tangible goals
After eight weeks of training, your targets will have shifted. Remember, tangible goals involve numbers and must be achievable and realistic. They don't have to be dramatic, just something that you can work toward steadily. For example, taking 30 seconds off your 5k time may not sound like a lot, but it would mean improvement of six seconds per kilometer. That would be a huge accomplishment.

Here are some "Beyond the 5k" tangible goal ideas:
- Run three days per week for four weeks
- Run a 5k in under X minutes
- Improve average 1km speed by Y seconds
- Participate in four 5k races over a season

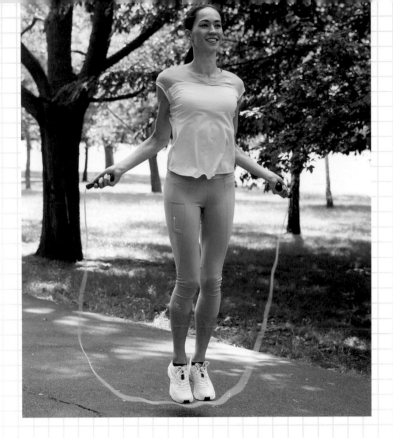

4 **Make time to train**
Just as you did in Warm-Up Week, get out your diary and plot those appointments with yourself. Get into a routine of doing this at the same time each week.

5 **Try something new**
Shake things up with a new route, a new running buddy, a new cross-training activity, or some new stickers for your training diary.

6 **Boost your support network**
Building a supportive running community is a great way to consolidate your new, healthy habits. We'll talk about how to do this next.

7 **Sign up for another race**
There's no better way to bring purpose to your workouts than having a race date in your calendar. It motivates you to train consistently so you'll be in good shape for the race and also gives you something to look forward to. Search for a race that inspires you in some way, whether it's an interesting location or a novelty theme. During your training you can visualize what fun you'll have, what you'll wear, how you'll run the race, and, of course, how you'll celebrate afterward!

Your motivation will evolve over time. It will ebb and flow according to your current family situation, career, and other priorities that affect your lifestyle. There will be highs and lows. But if you regularly revisit your motivation and make sure it still inspires you, create your goals, and plan to support that vision, your running will thrive.

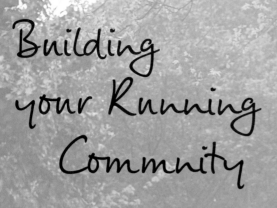

Building your Running Commnity

Chances are the first eight weeks of your running career were a solitary affair. Perhaps you wanted to keep your **running habit** quiet until you knew it was a keeper, or perhaps you just savored having regular time to yourself.

And that's fine—one of the best things about running is the quality alone time—just you, your thoughts, and the **open road**.

But as you consolidate your running habit and start to move beyond the 5k, it's a good idea to start building a running community. As great as it is to run alone, sharing the experience adds a new dimension to your training. Having a support network of fellow runners reminds you that you're a "real runner," and running is now a normal, everyday part of your life.

Whether you're an introvert or a social animal, you can build a community in a way that suits you. There are myriad "real world" and online options. See if any of these appeals to you.

Sign Up for More Races

As well as the training benefits we discussed earlier, one of the best things about racing is being part of a crowd of runners. Seeing the wide range of ages, sizes, and abilities always enforces the "if they can do it, I can do it!" spirit. It's also a great way to make friends. Julia met many of her regular running partners at local races. Be brave and strike up a conversation at the starting line—you could end up with a running date.

Running Clubs

No matter where you live, chances are your town or city has a local running club. Running clubs often have group workouts, local races, and social events. Check your local gyms, sport and recreation centers, or simply search online for "your town + running clubs."

Fellow Runners

Runners love any excuse to talk about running. And you'd be surprised how many people just want to help others, especially when you're tapping into something they're so passionate about. If you happen to know other runners, start a conversation. Don't worry if they have more running experience than you have. They'll just be overjoyed that someone else has joined the running fraternity.

Your Family and Friends...On Bikes

Julia's husband does not run. But he's still a great source of support for Julia. When she wants company on a long run, he follows her on his bicycle, chatting away as she does her various drills and intervals. It's a creative way to spend some time with loved ones with the added benefit of exercise.

Social Media

It's not just for cat videos and photos of your dinner. Posting your intention to run on your favorite network can be motivating, especially if your friends demand you post a red-faced selfie to prove you followed through. Social media is also a great source of inspiration—search the "running" hashtag on various social-media platforms for motivating quotes, photos, and links.

Online Running Forums

The forum has proved the most popular part of our Up & Running online courses. It's a thriving, supportive community with members from all over the globe. These connections have spilled into the real world, with members meeting up for races or even just coffee and cake. There are countless online running communities, such as those connected with running magazines or running apps, and most have free memberships.

Running Blogs

Whether they're written by a fellow novice or an élite athlete, running blogs are a great source of inspiration, information, and vicarious thrills. The highs and lows, race reports, and geeky running data all make for addictive reading. Many popular running blogs have lively communities in the comments sections. You could even start your own blog and share your journey.

Running Drills

These drills will build your strength and stamina and help you to run farther, faster.

Throughout the "Beyond the 5k" plans, you'll see the term "running in progression." It's an exercise that trains you to explore different speeds without pushing the gas pedal too hard. It helps you develop a sense of pacing so you can finish a race or workout strongly.

■ Start off running at a slow speed. How slow? Whatever "slow" feels like to you. This is a sensory workout just as much as it is aerobic. There is no "right" way to do it except to keep experimenting and gaining confidence in your running skills.

■ Gradually increase your speed, once, twice, or even three times. Think of it as shifting gears, moving from first, second, and then into third. The important thing is that you finish at a faster pace than you started.

■ Some workouts have a variation of this exercise: running in light progression. In this case, think of using two of your running gears and not reaching top speed.

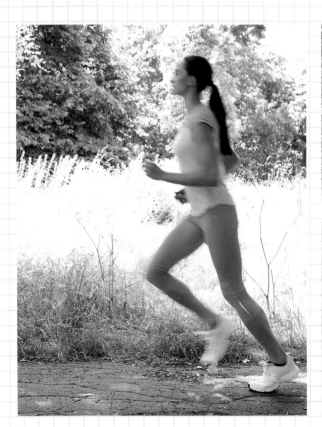
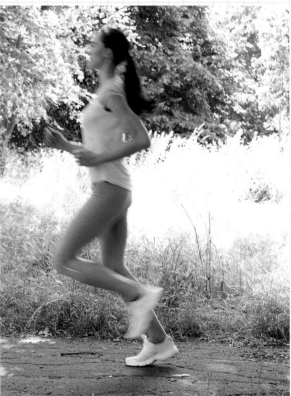

Sagittal Jumps

Sagittal jumps are a great exercise for strengthening quadriceps, glutes, and thigh flexors.
They also work your feet and ankles.

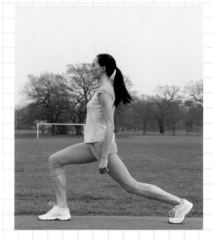 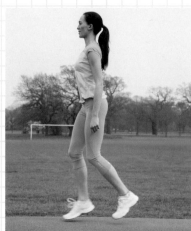 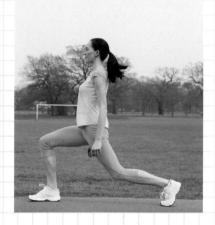

1 Start from a sagittal-split position by placing your left foot in front of you and your right foot behind.

2 Bend both knees, lower your body, and then take a quick jump, switching your foot position so you land with your right foot in front and your left foot behind. Keep your back straight and look forward as you jump.

3 Jump back and forth continuously until you've done a total of 12 jumps. This shouldn't take more than 15 seconds. The jumps will become easier once you gain some momentum.

Crunches

Strong abdominal muscles help you maintain good posture, which in turn allows you to run more efficiently.

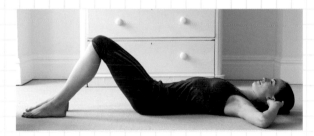 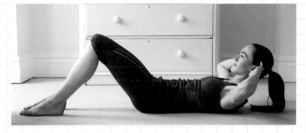

1 Lay down on a flat surface. Place your legs slightly apart. Leave your feet free. Don't have anybody sit on them or anchor them under a couch. This puts too much strain on your legs and hip-flexor muscles and doesn't target your abdominal muscles. Clasp your hands behind your head.

2 From a lying position, pull your torso toward your knees, exhaling as you come up. Concentrate on your abdominal muscles, feeling them tense as you rise. Stop when you're just a few inches off the ground. Hold the position just a second and then lower yourself back down and inhale.

High-Knee Runs

High-knee runs help develop muscular coordination and increase strength in your feet, legs, hips, and core.

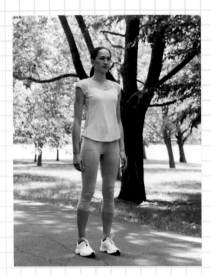 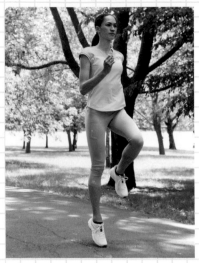 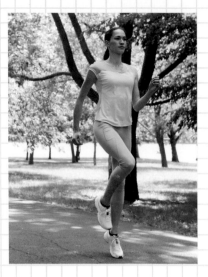

1 Keep your gaze forward with your head, back, and torso straight.

2 Coordinate your arms with your running steps. Keep your elbows at 90-degrees and use them to balance and push you forward.

3 Land and push off with your forefoot, never with your heels.

Small warning: High-knee runs are a difficult drill and require energy and concentration. If you're finding them difficult, you can start with forward-marching steps, then finish with high-knee runs. Try to do these runs on a soft surface to reduce impact.

Low-Knee Skipping

This is a variation of the skipping drill you did in the 5k program, except this time you don't lift your knees as high. Place more emphasis on your foot and ankle action and less on hips, quads, and hamstrings.

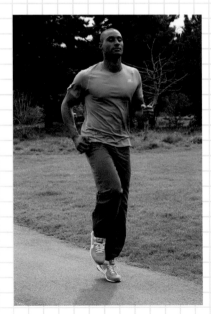 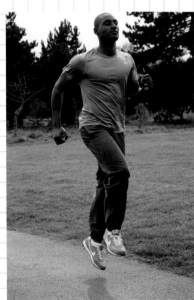

Strides

Strides are a basic running drill in which you run at a progressively faster speed over a short distance. It is not an all-out sprint. Performed correctly, strides will translate into faster, relaxed running at longer distances.

Break your stride into three sections:

- Start out slowly and progressively pick up your speed and rhythm to a fast, maximum speed.
- Maintain your speed while keeping your posture and form in check.
- Gradually slow down for the last third of the distance.

When you've finished the first stride exercise, take 40–60 seconds to catch your breath before you start the next one.

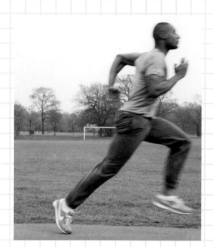
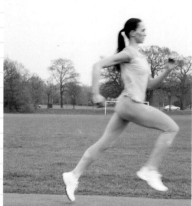

Uphill Strides

These short, maximum-intensity efforts against gravity help strengthen all your running muscles. They also increase the power and efficiency of flat strides, as you will be able to cover more ground with each stride using less energy.

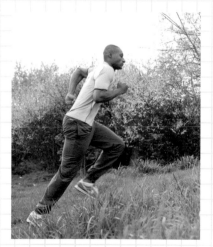
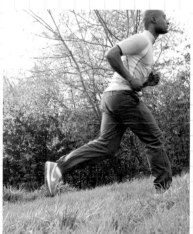
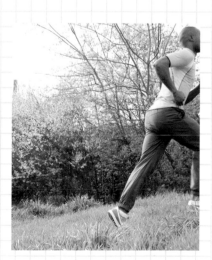

Find a slight incline; it doesn't need to be steep. Follow the same steps as flat strides. Recover by walking or slowly running back to your starting point After all, it's downhill.

Double Foot Hops

Think of foot hops as an advanced version of heel lifts.

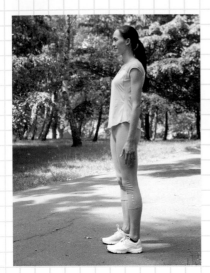 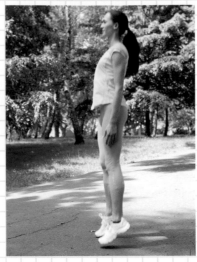

Do your hops in fast succession, pushing up and landing on the balls of your feet.

1 Stand on a flat surface with your knees locked out. You can either place your hands on your hips or simply relax your arms by your side.

2 Take a quick vertical hop by lifting both heels and pushing off the ground with the balls of your feet. You won't come off the ground more than half an inch.

Deep Breathing

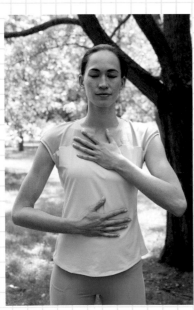

In order to run well, you need a nice flow of oxygen through your system. You might be thinking, "I'm alive and breathing, so oxygen is definitely flowing." But many runners take shallow breaths, only utilizing a small portion of their lung capacity. This can cause fatigue, side stitches, muscle cramps, and poor running performance.

Practice deep breathing with this exercise. Place one hand on your chest and the other on your belly. Breathe in deeply for three counts and exhale for two counts, pushing the air out of your lungs a little faster on the exhale. Feel your belly expanding more than your chest, which indicates that you're utilizing all your lung space and not just taking shallow breaths. Continue with this breathing pattern for two minutes. If you feel dizzy, it's the oxygen going to your head.

Beyond the 5k

Training Plans

The amazing thing about running is that you don't have to make drastic changes to improve your skills and conditioning. It's just a matter of varying your workouts in simple and subtle ways—changing speeds, taking less recovery time, adding a running drill.

That's how our three "Beyond the 5k" training plans bridge the gap between the 5k and 10k distance. "Aerobic Base Blast," "Running Style Revamp," and "Metabolism Mix Up" each have a specific workout theme and gently guide you through four weeks of training.

The first thing you'll notice about the "Beyond the 5k" plans is the weekly variety. You'll still be running three days a week, but while two of those workouts are the same, the third is different. You'll need around 45–50 minutes per workout. Remember, this is quality over quantity.

Choose your plan based on the guidelines at the start of this chapter, but feel free to mix and match the workouts to create your own. You'll be familiar with most of the running drills, but we've added in a few more to hone your running technique. Each plan also includes a circuit-training workout for total body conditioning.

As before for the 5k program, the possibility for treadmill modifications exists for all of these plans. Simply hop off the treadmill to do your stretches and non-running drills, such as skipping. But once again we encourage you to run outdoors to enjoy fully the variety and benefits of the training.

Plan 1
Aerobic Base Blast

Are you still gasping for breath throughout your workouts? Do you take lots of walking breaks during your Free Form Runs? This plan will help you keep building your fitness and get more comfortable with running for longer times and distances. You'll boost your results by running at a steady pace with a few faster intervals and drills thrown in.

Week 1

Workout 1

- Slow run — 10:00
- Stretch and deep breathing — 2:00
- 10 x (100m skip/50m recovery walk/50m jog)
- 3 x 7:00 run in light progression

1 **Slow run**
Warm up by running for 10 minutes at a slow pace.

2 **Stretch and deep breathing**
Stretch for a few minutes as you take in deep, intentional breaths.

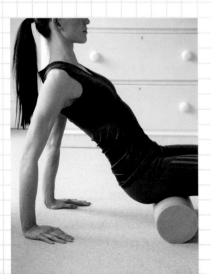

3 **10 x (100m skip/50m recovery walk/50m jog)**
Find a flat, even surface on which to skip for 100 meters. The distance does not have to be precise. Recover by walking back to the starting point for the first 50 meters and then slowly jog the last 50 meters. Repeat for a total of 10 times.

4 **3 x 7:00 run in light progression**
Each seven-minute block should be run in light progression, starting out at a slow and ending at a steady pace. There is no recovery here, simply run slowly for the first few minutes of each block and recover your breath before increasing your speed again.

Treadmill Modifications
- Thirty seconds of skipping equate to 100 meters.

Workout 2

- Slow run — 15:00
- Stretch — 2:00
- Run — 20:00 (10:00 at a slow pace/10:00 in light progression)

1 **Slow run**
Warm up by running for 15 minutes at a slow pace.

2 **Stretch**
Take two minutes for a good stretch.

3 **Run (10:00 at a slow pace/10:00 in light progression)**
Run for 20 minutes with the first 10 at an intentionally slow pace. Then run the last 10 in light progression without pushing yourself too hard.

Workout 3

Repeat Workout 1.

Week 2

Workout 1

- Slow run — 15:00
- Stretch — 2:00
- 5 x (50m uphill strides/ recovery walk back to start)
- Recovery walk — 5:00
- 5 x (100m strides/recovery walk back to start)
- Run — 20:00 (10:00 in light progression/10:00 at medium effort)

1 Slow run
Warm up by running for 15 minutes at a slow pace.

2 Stretch
Take two minutes for a good stretch.

3 5 x (50m uphill strides/ recovery walk back to start)
Find a slight uphill area. It doesn't need to be steep. As you start running uphill, remember to keep a steady, even leg turnover. Keep your arms at a 90-degree angle and use them in sync with your legs to help you push up the hill. Recover your energy by walking back down the hill to your starting point. Repeat four more times.

4 Recovery walk
Recover with a five-minute walk before going on to the next set of strides.

5 5 x (100m strides/ recovery walk back to start)
Choose a 100-meter distance with a flat, even surface. The measurement doesn't need to be precise. Progressively pick up your speed and cadence as you run each stride. Pay attention to your posture (back straight, shoulders relaxed) and arm position (elbows at a 90-degree angle). At the end of each set, walk back to your starting point and begin the next.

6 Run (10:00 in light progression/10:00 at medium effort)
These 20 minutes of running are broken into two parts. Begin the first 10 minutes with a slow run and progressively work up to a medium-effort pace. For the next 10 minutes, try and hold that same pace. Make sure the speed you choose is an effort you can sustain.

Treadmill Modifications
- Replace the uphill strides with 5 x 00:30 uphill walking on the treadmill, increasing the incline to 6 percent or more. Stop the treadmill between intervals and march in place for 30 seconds before starting the next one.
- Replace strides with 00:30 of running at a faster pace. Recover with 1:00 of slow walking.

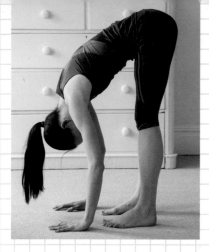

Workout 2

- Slow run — 10:00
- Stretch and deep breathing — 2:00
- 10 x (3:00 medium effort run/1:00 fast walk)

1 Slow run
Warm up by running for 10 minutes at a slow pace.

2 Stretch and deep breathing
Stretch for a few minutes as you take in deep, intentional breaths.

3 10 x (3:00 medium effort run/1:00 fast walk)
For a total of 40 minutes, alternate three minutes of running with one minute recovery walking. Medium effort is a speed you can sustain for the whole workout. Slow down if you find that one minute walking is not enough time to recover from the run segments.

Workout 3

Repeat Workout 1.

Week 3

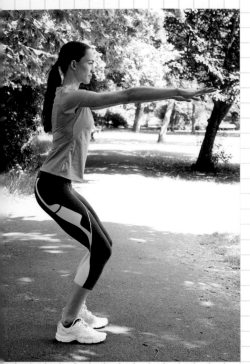

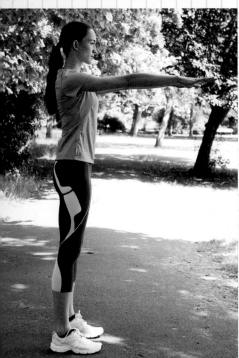

Workout 1

- Slow run — 20:00
- Circuit training: 3 x (5 half squats/2:00 medium effort run/6 sagittal jumps/ 1:00 fast walk with arm windmills/10 heel lifts/ 100m skip/10 crunches/ 1km slow run)

1 Slow run
Warm up by running for 20 minutes at a slow pace.

2 Circuit training
This circuit involves five exercises interspersed with running and walking. Do each exercise in sequence, flowing from one to the next without pause.

- Begin with five half squats.
- Follow with a two-minute run at medium effort.
- Now stop and perform six sagittal jumps per leg.
- Follow with a one-minute walk at fast pace as you perform arm windmills.
- Stop to do 10 heel lifts and then continue with 100 meters of skipping.
- Hit the ground for 10 crunches.
- Finish with a 1km slow run.
- You can take a minute to recover between each circuit if necessary.

Workout 2

- Slow run — 10:00
- 3 x (10:00 run in light progression/1:00 recovery walk)

1 Slow run
Warm up by running for 10 minutes at a slow pace.

2 3 x (10:00 run in light progression/1:00 recovery walk)
Think of this main running segment as a roller coaster for your heart rate. Begin each 10-minute segment of running with slow running and gradually work your way up to a fast pace. Recover with a one-minute walk to get your breathing and heart rate under control and then finish off the workout with two more 10-minute progressions.

Workout 3

Repeat Workout 1.

Week 4

Workout 1

- Slow run — 15:00
- 5 x 100m strides
- 5 x (3:00 medium-fast effort run/3:00 recovery walk) — 30:00
- Slow cool-down run — 5:00

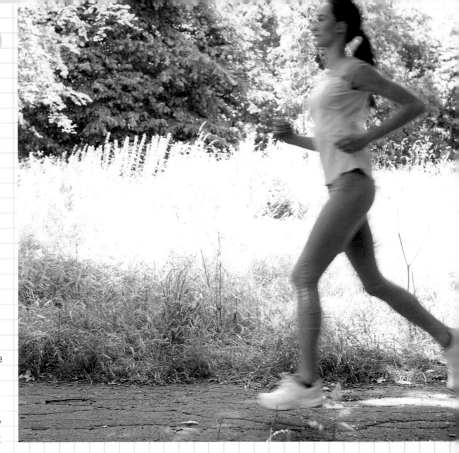

1 Slow run
Warm up by running for 15 minutes at a slow pace.

2 5 x 100m strides
Choose a 100-meter distance with a flat, even surface. The measurement doesn't need to be exact. As you run each stride, progressively pick up your speed and cadence. Pay attention to your posture and arm position by making sure your back is straight and arms are relaxed at a 90-degree angle. At the end of each set, take a 30-second break before starting the next one.

Treadmill Modifications
- Replace strides with 00:30 of running at a faster pace. Recover with 1:00 of slow walking.

3 5 x (3:00 medium-fast effort run/3:00 recovery walk)
Choose a running speed that you can sustain for three minutes, but fast enough that you'll need three more recovery minutes of walking. Alternate between the medium-fast run and the recovery walk for a total of 30 minutes.

4 Slow cool-down run
Cool down by running for five minutes at a slow pace.

Workout 2

- 2 x (20:00 even effort run/ 5:00 recovery walk)

For your first 20-minute running segment, find a pace that you feel is comfortable. Try to keep the speed steady and even. After 20 minutes, take a five-minute walking break. Finish the workout with another 20 minutes of running.

Workout 3

Repeat Workout 1.

Plan 2
Running Style Revamp

Can you hear your feet shuffling while you run? Are you at an average weight, running the entire Free Form Running segments but still not obtaining the times you want? The problem is most likely found in your running style and mechanics. Running Style Revamp features more advanced versions of the drills you know from the 5k program.

Week 1

Workout 1

- Slow run — 10:00
- Deep-breathing exercise — 2:00
- 5 x (100m skip/50m recovery walk/50m run)
- 5 x 50m knee-high runs
- 4 x 6:00 run in light progression — 24:00

1 **Slow run**
Warm up by running for 10 minutes at a slow pace.

2 **Deep-breathing exercise**
Place one hand on your chest and the other on your belly. Breathe in deeply for three counts and exhale for two, pushing the air out of your lungs a little faster on the exhale. Breathe through either your nose or mouth. Feel your belly expanding more than your chest, which indicates you're using all your lung capacity and not just taking shallow breaths. Continue this breathing pattern for two minutes.

3 **5 x (100m skip/50m recovery walk/50m run)**
Choose a 100-meter distance with a flat, even surface. The measurement doesn't need to be precise. As you skip, concentrate on using your feet to push yourself forward. Remember that your knees don't need to come up high. Walk back to the start for the first 50 meters and then break into a slow run for the remaining 50 meters. Repeat four more times.

4 **5 x 50m knee-high runs**
On the same even surface, guesstimate 50 meters and begin your knee-high runs. Concentrate on moving forward as your knees move up and down. Bend your elbows and use your arms for balance and propulsion. Take about 30 seconds to recover between each run. Complete five of these before moving on to the next segment.

5 **4 x 6:00 run in light progression**
Begin with slow running and work your way up to a fast pace. There is no walking recovery so make sure you start very slowly. Repeat these progressions four times for a total of 24 minutes.

Workout 2

- Slow run — 15:00
- Stretch — 5:00
- Run in light progression — 20:00

1 **Slow warm up run**
Warm up by running for 15 minutes at a slow pace.

2 **Stretch**
Take five minutes to stretch.

3 **Run in light progression**
We suggest 10 minutes at a slow speed, eight minutes at a moderate speed, and two minutes at a fast yet sustainable speed. Give it all you've got for those last two minutes because after that, you're all done.

Workout 3

Repeat Workout 1.

Treadmill Modifications
- Find a space near the treadmill for the skipping drill. Thirty seconds of skipping equate to 100 meters.
- Fifteen seconds are equivalent to 50 meters.

Week 2

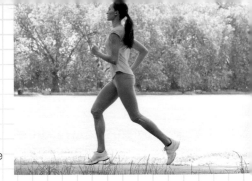

Workout 1

- Slow run — 15:00
- Stretch — 3:00
- 5 x (50m uphill strides/ recovery walk back to start)
- Recovery — 2:00
- 5 x (100m regular strides/ recovery walk back to start)
- 3 x (10 double foot hops in place/1:00 slow run)
- Run — 20:00

1 Slow run
Warm up by running for 15 minutes at a slow pace.

2 Stretch
Take three minutes for a good stretch.

3 5 x (50m uphill strides/ recovery walk back to start)
Find a slight uphill area. It doesn't need to be steep. As you start running uphill, remember to keep a steady, even leg turnover. Keep your arms at a 90-degree angle and use them in sync with your legs to help you push up the hill. Recover your energy by walking back down the hill to your starting point. Repeat four more times.

4 Recovery
Take two minutes to get your breathing under control. You can use this time to stretch again.

5 5 x (100m regular strides/recovery walk back to start)
Choose a 100-meter distance with a flat, even surface. Progressively pick up your speed and cadence, making sure your back is straight and your arms are relaxed at a 90-degree angle. At the end of each set, walk back to your starting point to recover before you start the next one.

6 3 x (10 double foot hops in place/1:00 slow run)
Foot hops are an advanced version of heel lifts. Stand on a flat surface with your knees locked. Take a quick vertical jump by lifting your heels and pushing off the ground with the balls of your feet. You won't come off the ground more than half an inch. Do 10 hops in fast succession then run slowly for one minute. Repeat two more times.

7 Run
Finish with a 20-minute run at an easy, relaxed pace.

Treadmill Modifications

- Replace the uphill strides with 5 x 00:30 uphill walking on the treadmill, increasing the incline to 6 percent or more. Stop the treadmill between intervals and march in place for 30 seconds before starting the next one.
- Replace strides with 00:30 of running at a faster pace. Recover with 1:00 of slow walking.

Workout 2

- 8 x (1:00 slow run/1:00 skip)
- Stretch — 5:00
- 10 x (3:00 steady effort run/1:00 fast recovery walk)

1 8 x (1:00 slow run/ 1:00 skip)
Alternate one minute of running with one minute of skipping. Repeat this cycle for a total of 16 minutes.

2 Stretch
Take a full five minutes for a good stretch, especially those calf muscles after the skipping.

3 10 x (3:00 steady effort run/1:00 fast recovery walk)
Run for three minutes at a steady pace and effort. Take a one-minute walking break, but remember to keep it fast. Repeat this cycle 10 times for a total of 40 minutes.

Workout 3

Repeat Workout 1.

Week 3

Workout 1

- Slow run — 20:00
- Circuit training: 3 x (5 half squats/2:00 medium effort run/6 sagittal jumps/1:00 fast walk with arm windmills/10 heel lifts/100m skip/10 crunches/1km slow run)

1 Slow run
Warm up by running for 20 minutes at a slow pace.

2 Circuit training
This circuit involves five exercises interspersed by running and walking. Do each exercise in sequence, flowing from one to the next without pause.

- Begin with five half squats.
- Follow with a two-minute run at medium effort.
- Now stop and perform six sagittal jumps per leg.
- Follow with a one-minute walk at fast pace as you perform arm windmills.
- Stop to do 10 heel lifts and then continue with 100 meters of skipping.
- Hit the ground for 10 crunches.
- Finish with a 1km slow run.
- You can take a minute to recover between each circuit if necessary.

Workout 2

- Run in light progression — 40:00

We suggest 20 minutes at a slow speed, 15 minutes at a moderate speed, and five minutes at a faster yet sustainable speed. This is "light" progression so it doesn't have to be an all-out effort.

Workout 3

Repeat Workout 1.

Week 4

Workout 1

- Slow run — 15:00
- 5 x (100m strides/recovery walk to start)
- 5 x (3:00 fast effort run/3:00 recovery walk)
- Slow cool-down run — 5:00

1 Slow run
Warm up by running for 15 minutes at a slow pace.

2 5 x (100m strides/recovery walk to start)
Choose a 100-meter distance with a flat, even surface. Progressively pick up your speed and cadence, making sure your back is straight and your arms are relaxed at a 90-degree angle. At the end of each set, walk back to your starting point to recover before you start the next one.

3 5 x (3:00 fast effort run/3:00 recovery walk)
Start running at a fast pace you feel you can maintain for the full three minutes. Recover for another three minutes by stretching or walking around. Repeat four more times for a total time of 30 minutes.

4 Slow cool-down run
Cool down with an easy five-minute run.

Workout 2

- Run — 40:00 (10:00 easy run/30:00 steady effort)

Run for a full 40 minutes, beginning with a 10-minute easy run to warm up and then ease into a steady effort and pace for the rest of your workout.

Workout 3

Repeat Workout 1.

Treadmill Modifications
- Replace strides with 00:30 of running at a faster pace. Recover with 1:00 of slow walking.

Plan 3
Metabolism Mix Up

Is your current body composition keeping you from running your best? Have you been on a fat-loss plateau for the last month even with your best efforts? This plan will help fire up your metabolism and improve your fitness. For an extra boost, add in one or two weekly cross-training workouts, each a minimum of 40 minutes. Try something different each week, but remember that an old-fashioned walk is always a great choice. Remember—to improve body composition you'll also need to follow a nutrition plan that supports your fitness activity.

Week 1

Workout 1

- Slow run — 10:00
- Deep-breathing exercise — 2:00
- 10 x (100m strides/100m recovery fast walk)
- 5 x 50m knee lifts marching forward
- 4 x (6:00 run/1:00 walk)

1 Slow run
Warm up by running for 10 minutes at a slow pace.

2 Deep-breathing exercise
Place one hand on your chest and the other on your belly. Breathe in deeply for three counts and exhale for two, pushing the air out a little faster on the exhale. Feel your belly expanding more than your chest, which indicates you're using all your lung capacity and not just taking shallow breaths. Continue this breathing pattern for two minutes.

3 10 x (100m strides/100m recovery fast walk)
Choose a 100-meter distance with a flat, even surface. Progressively pick up your speed and cadence, making sure your back is straight and your arms are relaxed at a 90-degree angle. At the end of each set, walk fast back to your starting point to start the next one.

4 5 x 50m knee lifts marching forward
This is a gentle way to activate those running-specific muscles without bouncing around. March forward for 50 meters on a flat and even surface. Lift your knees to about a 90-degree angle; they don't need to touch your chest. Take a minute's break between each interval.

5 4 x (6:00 run/1:00 walk)
Your main workout today is six minutes of running with a one-minute walk break, repeated four times for a total of 28 minutes. Your running pace and speed should be enjoyable and relaxing. Find your groove.

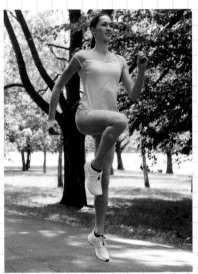

Treadmill Modifications
- Replace strides with 00:30 of running at a faster pace. Recover with 1:00 of slow walking.
- Slow the treadmill down to a walking pace for the knee lifts.

Workout 2

- Slow run — 20:00
- Stretch — 5:00
- Run in light progression — 20:00

1 Slow run
Warm up by running for 20 minutes at a slow pace.

2 Stretch
Take five minutes for a good stretch.

3 Run in light progression
This is a light progression so you should not go all out. Simply gradually increase your speed throughout the 20 minutes, but stay well within your comfort zone.

Workout 3

Repeat Workout 1.

Week 2

Workout 1

- Fast walk — 15:00
- Slow run — 15:00
- 5 x (100m strides/recovery walk back to start)
- 5 x (50m low-knee skip/ recovery walk back to start)
- Run in light progression — 15:00

1 Fast walk
Begin with fast walking. Increase your cadence and shorten your stride to gain a little speed.

2 Slow run
Continue your warm-up by breaking into a slow run for 15 minutes.

3 5 x (100m strides/ recovery walk back to start)
Choose a 100-meter distance with a flat, even surface. Progressively pick up your speed and cadence, making sure your back is straight and your arms are relaxed at a 90-degree angle. At the end of each set, walk back to your starting point to recover before you start the next one.

4 5 x (50m low-knee skip/ recovery walk back to start)
Keep your knees low as you move forward. Actively use your forefoot to push off the ground. For recovery, walk back to your starting point and then do four more rounds.

5 Run in light progression
Run in light progression for 15 minutes. "Light" means you don't need to go all out. Gradually increase your speed throughout the 15 minutes but stay well within your comfort zone.

Treadmill Modifications
- Replace strides with 00:30 of running at a faster pace. Recover with 1:00 of slow walking.

Workout 2

- Slow run — 10:00
- Fast walk — 5:00
- Steady effort run — 10:00
- Stretch — 5:00
- 10 x (1:00 steady effort run/ 1:00 slow run) — 20:00

1 Slow run
Warm up by running for 10 minutes at a slow pace.

2 Fast walk
Walk at a fast pace for five minutes.

3 Steady effort run
Begin running again but choose a speed somewhere between your slow pace and your medium pace. Concentrate on keeping that same steady effort for a full 10 minutes.

4 Stretching
Take a full five minutes for a good stretch.

5 10 x (1:00 steady effort run/1:00 slow run)
This last running segment is 20-minutes long, alternating between a slow run and a faster, steady run. The actual speed doesn't matter, just make sure that there is a perceived difference between the two.

Workout 3

Repeat Workout 1.

Week 3

Workout 1

- Slow run — 20:00
- Circuit training: 3 x (5 half squats/2:00 medium effort run/6 sagittal jumps/1:00 fast walk with arm windmills/10 heel lifts/100m skip/10 crunches/1km slow run)

1 Slow run
Begin your workout by warming up with an easy, slow-paced run for 20 minutes.

2 Circuit training
This circuit involves five exercises interspersed by running and walking. Do each exercise in sequence, flowing from one to the next without pause.

- Begin with five half squats.
- Follow with a two-minute run at medium effort.
- Now stop and perform six sagittal jumps per leg.
- Follow with a one-minute walk at fast pace as you perform arm windmills.
- Stop to do 10 heel lifts and then continue with a 100 meters of skipping.
- Hit the ground for 10 crunches.
- Finish with a 1km slow run.
- You can take a minute to recover between each circuit if necessary.

Workout 2

- Run in light progression — 40:00

Start off at a slow pace for at least the first 15 minutes. Gradually increase your speed throughout the last 30 minutes. "Light" means that you don't have to finish at a top speed, just faster than your starting speed.

Workout 3

Repeat Workout 1.

Week 4

Workout 1

- Slow run — 15:00
- 5 x (100m strides/recovery walk back to start)
- 6 x (4:00 steady effort run/1:00 run, concentrating on breathing) — 30:00
- Cool-down run — 5:00

1 Slow run
Begin your workout with a 15-minute warm-up run at an easy pace.

2 5 x 100m strides/recovery walk back to start)
Choose a 100-meter distance with a flat, even surface. Progressively pick up your speed and cadence, making sure your back is straight and your arms are relaxed at a 90-degree angle.

At the end of each set, walk back to your starting point to recover before you start the next one.

3 6 x (4:00 steady effort run/1:00 run while concentrating on breathing)
Run for a total of 30 minutes at steady effort (not too slow, not too fast). Every four minutes concentrate for 60 seconds on how you're breathing. Many new runners take shallow breaths so now is the time to practice taking deep and intentional ones.

4 Cool-down run
Take five minutes to cool down with a slow-paced run.

Workout 2

- 45:00 continuous run (15:00 easy/30:00 steady effort)

Think of this as a simple 45-minute run divided into two parts. Warm up for 15 minutes at a slow, easy pace. Increase your speed slightly for the last 30 minutes, running at a nice clip but not overexerting yourself.

Workout 3

Repeat Workout 1.

Treadmill Modifications
- Replace strides with 00:30 of running at a faster pace. Recover with 1:00 of slow walking.

Epilogue

"When you put yourself on the line in a race and expose yourself to the unknown, you learn things about yourself that are very exciting." DORIS BROWN HERITAGE

Running has always been more than a workout for us. We've guided thousands of people through the eight-week training plan and watched them emerge with not only stronger legs but a whole new perspective on themselves and their lives.

It's as if once they've conquered a goal that they thought was impossible, they look at the rest of their lives and wonder what other great things they could do. Suddenly anything feels possible.

Take the courage that you found with your running and apply it to your other dreams: longer races, bucket-list wishes, career ambitions. As long as you've got strong goals, a solid plan, and know your deepest motivations, you can take your life in so many new directions.

Here's to a future filled with all kinds of finish lines.

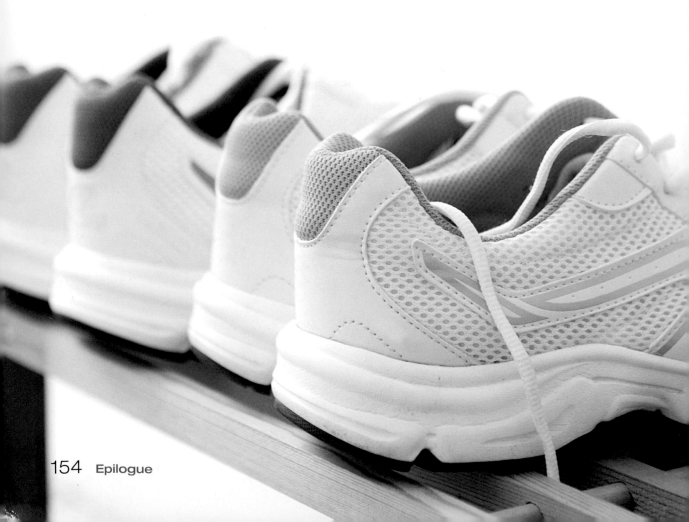

Resources

Find a Race

- **Runners World:** comprehensive race listings, *runnersworld.com/races-places*
- **Active:** global race finder, *active.com*
- **Race for the Cure:** worldwide series of charity 5k races, *raceforthecure.org*
- **Race for Life:** UK series of charity 5k races, *raceforlife.cancerresearchuk.org*
- **Parkrun:** free, timed weekly 5k runs, *parkrun.com*

Apps and Websites

- **Up & Running:** running tips and inspiration from your authors, *upandrunningonline.org*
- **Runkeeper:** Android and iPhone app for runners, *runkeeper.com*
- **Runmeter:** iPhone app for tracking workouts, *abvio.com/runmeter*
- **MapMyRun:** measure and map your running routes, *mapmyrun.com*
- **Gmap Pedometer:** free site for mapping routes, *gmap-pedometer.com*
- **Headspace:** includes a free 10-day meditation program, *getsomeheadspace.com*
- **Buddhify2:** packed with meditations for different situations and times of day, *buddhify.com*

- **You Are Your Own Gym:** great app with bodyweight exercises, *marklauren.com/apps.html*
- **Yoga Studio:** free yoga classes on your phone, *yogastudioapp.com*

Running Blogs

- **Ask Lauren Fleshman:** journal of professional runner, *asklaurenfleshman.com*
- **Shut Up & Run:** humor, tips, and inspiration from Beth, *shutupandrun.net*
- **Steve In A Speedo:** hilarious tales from a Minnesotan runner and triathlete, *iwannagetphysical.blogspot.com*
- **Meals and Miles:** Meghann writes about food and running, *mealsandmiles.com*
- **She Climbed Until She Saw:** Lori lost 210 pounds and became a runner, *intheequation.com*

Podcasts

- **Marathon Talk:** don't be put off by the "M" word, this podcast is inspiring for all levels and features interviews with running legends, *marathontalk.com*
- **Jillian Michaels:** inspiration, advice, and laughs from the famous trainer, *jillianmichaels.com*
- **Trail Runner Nation:** great expert interviews and inspiration if you love being in the great outdoors, *trailrunnernation.com*

- **Fitness Behavior:** explores the behaviors and habits that lead to fitness success, *bevanjameseyles.com/fitness-behavior*

Sportswear

USA

- **Road Runner Sports:** "the world's largest running & walking store," *roadrunnersports.com*
- **Amazon:** find last season's running shoes at bargain prices, *amazon.com*
- **Walmart:** stocks Danskin sportswear up to size 2X, *walmart.com*
- **Target:** great range of affordable sportswear, *target.com*
- **Oiselle:** up and coming independent sportswear brand, *oiselle.com*
- **Lululemon:** pricey but gorgeous running gear, *lululemon.com*

UK

- **Decathlon:** a huge range of shoes and sportswear, *decathlon.com*
- **Wiggle:** comprehensive online sports retailer, includes running and cycling gear, *wiggle.co.uk*
- **Less Bounce:** sports bras for chests of all sizes. UK site with international shipping, *lessbounce.com*

Weekly Training Diaries

Week 1

Workout	Date	1km walk (MM:ss)	1km Free Form Run (MM:ss)	Total workout time (MM:ss)	Estimated total distance	Notes
1		:	:	:		
2		:	:	:		
3		:	:	:		

Weekly stats   Total workout time this week: .... Estimated total distance this week: ....

Week 2

Workout	Date	1km Free Form Run (MM:ss)	Total workout time (MM:ss)	Estimated total distance	Notes
1		:	:		
2		:	:		
3		:	:		

Weekly stats   Total workout time this week: .... Estimated total distance this week: ....

Week 3

Workout	Date	1km Free Form Run 1 (MM:ss)	1km Free Form Run 2 (MM:ss)	Total workout time (MM:ss)	Estimated total distance	Notes
1		:	:	:		
2		:	:	:		
3		:	:	:		

Weekly stats   Total workout time this week: .... Estimated total distance this week: ....

Week 4

Workout	Date	1.5km Free Form Run (MM:ss)	Total workout time (MM:ss)	Estimated total distance	Notes
1		:	:		
2		:	:		
3		:	:		

Weekly stats   Total workout time this week: .... Estimated total distance this week: ....

Week 5

Workout	Date	1km Free Form Run (MM:ss)	Total workout time (MM:ss)	Estimated total distance	Notes
1		:	:		
2		:	:		
3		:	:		

Weekly stats   Total workout time this week: ....   Estimated total distance this week: ....

Week 6

Workout	Date	1km Free Form Run 1 (MM:ss)	1km Free Form Run 2 (MM:ss)	1km Free Form Run 3 (MM:ss)	Total workout time (MM:ss)	Estimated total distance	Notes
1		:	:	:	:		
2		:	:	:	:		
3		:	:	:	:		

Weekly stats   Total workout time this week: ....   Estimated total distance this week: ....

Week 7

Workout	Date	2km Free Form Run (MM:ss)	1km Free Form Run (MM:ss)	Total workout time (MM:ss)	Estimated total distance	Notes
1		:	:	:		
2		:	:	:		
3		:	:	:		

Weekly stats   Total workout time this week: ....   Estimated total distance this week: ....

Week 8

Workout	Date	2km Free Form Run (MM:ss)	1km Free Form Run #1 (MM:ss)	1km Free Form Run #2 (MM:ss)	Total workout time (MM:ss)	Estimated total distance	Notes
1		:	:	:	:		
2		:	:	:	:		
3*					:	5km	

Weekly stats   Total workout time this week: ....   Estimated total distance this week: ....

* Your 5k race

Index

Acknowledgments

Thank you to our wonderful Up & Running athletes. We've learned so much from you all, both personally and professionally. You bring so much sparkle to this book and to our lives!

We would also like to thank Lauren Mulholland for her smart and thoughtful editing and for the opportunity to make our book dream a reality.

Julia
My thanks to Piero, Evan, and Olivia for their endless love and support in following my dreams. Special thanks to Shauna without whom Up & Running would not exist...here's to more dreaming in Amsterdam.

Shauna
Thank you to my friends and family for your support and patience while writing this book, especially to Gareth, Rhiannon, and The Mothership. Special shout out to Apple's voice dictation software, and to Julia Jones for inspiring me every day with your grace, wisdom, and amazing athletic feats.